THE ROLE OF LUTEINIZING HORMONE IN FOLLICULOGENESIS AND OVULATION INDUCTION

Editor
MARCO FILICORI
Reproductive Endocrinology Center
University of Bologna

MONDUZZI EDITORE

Monduzzi Editore S.p.A., via Ferrarese, 119/2 - 40128 Bologna - Italy
Phone (+) 39-051-4151123 - Fax (+) 39-051-4151125

Printed in February 1999 by Litosei - Rastignano - Bologna (Italy)

Index

Principal Contributors

D.R. Danforth
Department of Obstetrics and Gynecology
The Ohio State University
5th Fl Means Hl
1654 Upham Dr
Columbus, OH 43210-1228
USA

K. Diedrich
Klinik für Frauenheilkunde und Geburtshilfe
Medizinische Universität zu Lübeck
Ratzeburger Allee 160
D-23538 Lübeck
GERMANY

M. Filicori
Reproductive Endocrinology Center
University of Bologna
Via Massarenti, 13
40138 Bologna
ITALY

R. Fleming
University Department of Obstetrics and Gynecology
Royal Infirmary
10 Alexandra Parade
Glasgow G31 2ER
UNITED KINGDOM

U. Gordon
Center for Reproductive Medicine
4 Priory Road
Clifton, Bristol BS8 1TY
UNITED KINGDOM

S.G. Hillier
Reproductive Medicine Laboratory
University of Edinburgh
Centre for Reproductive Biology
37 Chalmers St.
Edinburgh EH3 9EW
UNITED KINGDOM

R. Homburg
Department of Obstetrics & Gynecology
Golda Medical Center (Hasharon)
49372 Petah Tikva
ISRAEL

A. Lanzone
Clinica Ostetrica e Ginecologica
Policlinico "A. Gemelli"
Largo A. Gemelli 8
00168 Roma
ITALY

N.S. Macklon
Section Reproductive Endocrinology
Department of Obstetrics and Gynecology
Dijkzigt Academy Hospital
3015 Rotterdam
THE NETHERLANDS

R. Quinton
Department of Endocrinology
Cobbold Laboratories
The Middlesex Hospital
Mortimer Street
London W1N 8AA
UNITED KINGDOM

Z. Shoham
Department of Obstetrics &
Gynecology
Kaplan Hospital
Rehovot 76100
ISRAEL

L.G. Westergaard
Fertility Clinic
Department of Obstetrics and
Ginecology
Odense University Hospital
DK 5000 Odense C
DENMARK

A.J. Zeleznik
Department of Obstetrics and
Gynecology
Magee-Womens Research Institute
204 Craft Ave, Room 524
Pittsburgh, PA 15213
USA

M.B. Zelinski-Wooten
Oregon Regional Primate
Research Center
505 NW 185th Avenue
Beaverton, OR 97006
USA

Foreword

For many decades we have known that pituitary gonadotropins, both follicle stimulating hormone (FSH) and luteinizing hormone (LH), are in control of menstrual cycle dynamics and ovulation. Over three decades ago the introduction of medications that were capable of inducing ovarian function through indirect (clomiphene citrate) or direct (menotropins) gonadotropin stimulation revolutionized treatment of reproductive disorders in women and men.

Until the early 1980s human menotropin preparations contained comparable amounts of LH and FSH; however, in the last 15 years new drugs with progressively lower amounts of LH activity were made available for the treatment of anovulation and for controlled ovarian stimulation in assisted reproduction. At the same time, the introduction of gonadotropin releasing hormone (GnRH) agonists optimized assisted reproduction regimens but also further reduced overall ovarian LH stimulation. In the near future the association of recombinant human FSH and GnRH antagonists may result in stimulatory regimens virtually devoid of LH activity.

In physiological circumstances LH and FSH can be seen as a team collaborating for the achievement of a common goal, the maturation and ovulation of reproductively competent oocytes. Does the same principle apply to ovulation induction? The logical corollary to this question is whether or not LH stimulation is of any practical value in ovulation induction regimens. These issues are being raised increasingly more often by both investigators and clinicians and are of the utmost scientific and medical value. Optimization of ovulation induction regimens can significantly reduce overall costs of already very expensive assisted reproduction procedures and limit sacrifices and complications imposed upon our patients.

This volume contains all the scientific contributions presented at the Workshop "The Role of Luteinizing Hormone in Folliculogenesis and Ovulation Induction" that was held in Bologna, Italy on October 30-31, 1998.

This meeting was organized to provide basic and therapeutic answers to questions related to the physiologic, pathophysiologic and clinical role of LH in female reproduction. Thanks to the excellent quality of presentations and the interest of these issues this meeting was attended by over 240 scientists and clinicians from all over the world.

I wish to take this opportunity to thank the Speakers for their outstanding contributions and timely manuscript submission that allowed a rapid publication of these proceedings, Dr. Gabriella Benassi of S.P. International for flawless organizational support, and Ralph Diehl, Sean Davis, and Anja Lindner of Ferring GmbH for believing in the concept of this workshop.

I hope that you will enjoy reading this book as much as did and that the information contained in this volume will help in stimulating debate and further research in this critical area of reproductive endocrinology.

Marco Filicori, MD

Bologna, January 1999

The Role of Luteinizing Hormone
in Folliculogenesis
and Ovulation Induction, pp. 1-19
Editor M. Filicori

Gonadotropic Control of Follicular Development in Primates

A.J. Zeleznik and M.W. Sullivan

Departments of Cell Biology and Physiology (AJZ) and
Obstetrics, Gynecology and Reproductive Sciences (AJZ, MWS)
University of Pittsburgh School of Medicine, Pittsburgh, PA (United States of America)

Abstract. *During the follicular phase of the menstrual cycle of human and subhuman primates, a single follicle is selected to mature and release its oocyte for ovulation and potential fertilization. Previous studies in both humans and nonhuman primates have demonstrated that follicle stimulating hormone (FSH) is absolutely required for the initiation of follicular development and estrogen production. It is also now well established that the absolute concentrations of FSH achieved during the follicular phase of the menstrual cycle are responsible not only for the initiation of follicular growth but also for the selective maturation of a single preovulatory follicle. Thus, in order for preovulatory follicular growth to commence, serum FSH concentrations must surpass a critical "threshold" level. Once threshold levels of FSH are achieved, large preantral follicles are stimulated to grow and produce estrogen. If FSH levels are maintained above threshold levels, multiple follicles will mature to the preovulatory stage. However, during the spontaneous follicular phase, the secretion of estrogen by the maturing follicle suppresses FSH secretion below the critical threshold levels and the maturation of other less mature follicles is curtailed leading to a monotocous ovulation.*

While the aforementioned mechanism for follicle selection is well established both experimentally and clinically, a complete solution to the problem of follicle selection must include an explanation as to how the maturing follicle is spared from its self-imposed reduction of serum FSH concentrations. This goal of this chapter is to summarize the current knowledge regarding the process of follicle selection during the menstrual cycle with particular emphasis on the cellular and physiological mechanisms by which the maturing follicle is spared from the decline in plasma FSH concentrations during the mid through late follicular phase.

Key words. Follicle selection, follicle stimulating hormone, luteinizing hormone, hormone receptors, angiogenesis.

Introduction

In 1943 the late Roy Greep and co-workers[1] were the first to separate and purify two distinct anterior pituitary gonadotropins which they called thylakentrin (FSH) and metakentrin (LH). They further demonstrated in hypophysectomized rats that while FSH was able to stimulate the appearance of antral follicles, the ability of these hypophysectomized animals to produce estrogen and form corpora lutea was dependent upon stimulation by both FSH and LH. In the 1950's and 1960's the demonstrations that ovulation could be restored in gonadotropin-deficient monkeys and humans with exogenous FSH and LH[2-4] led to the wide spread use of gonadotropin therapy to restore ovulation in anovulatory women as well as to produce multiple oocytes for fertilization in assisted reproduction procedures. Despite the clinical use of gonadotropins for over thirty years, the physiological mechanisms by which a single preovulatory follicle is formed each menstrual cycle has yet to be elucidated. Moreover, the use of exogenous gonadotropins to stimulate ovulation in women is frequently accompanied by the undesired complication of multiple follicular maturation and ovarian hyperstimulation syndrome. The goal of this chapter is to summarize the extant knowledge regarding the individual roles of FSH and LH in the process of follicular development and to provide new insights as to how these hormones may interact with the ovary to produce a single preovulatory during the spontaneous menstrual cycle.

Gonadotropins and follicular development

The use of surface binding autoradiography by Midgley and co-workers[5] to identify the cell types within the ovary that contain receptors for FSH and LH as well as tissue culture studies with isolated theca and granulosa cells[6,7] provided the analytical resources for the elucidation the physiological effects of the gonadotropins on ovarian cellular function. Figure 1 summarizes the distribution of gonadotropin receptors and steroidogenic enzymes in immature and preovulatory follicles.

FSH. Studies using autoradiography demonstrated that receptors for FSH were confined specifically to the granulosa cells of follicles while LH receptors were uniformly present on theca cells of follicles[5]. This observation was somewhat perplexing because it was well established that LH is the principal hormone involved in the transformation of the follicle into a corpus luteum yet granulosa cells, the precursor cells of the corpus luteum, did not possess LH receptors. The observations by Channing and Kammerman[8] that LH receptors are absent on granulosa cells isolated from small follicles but are present on

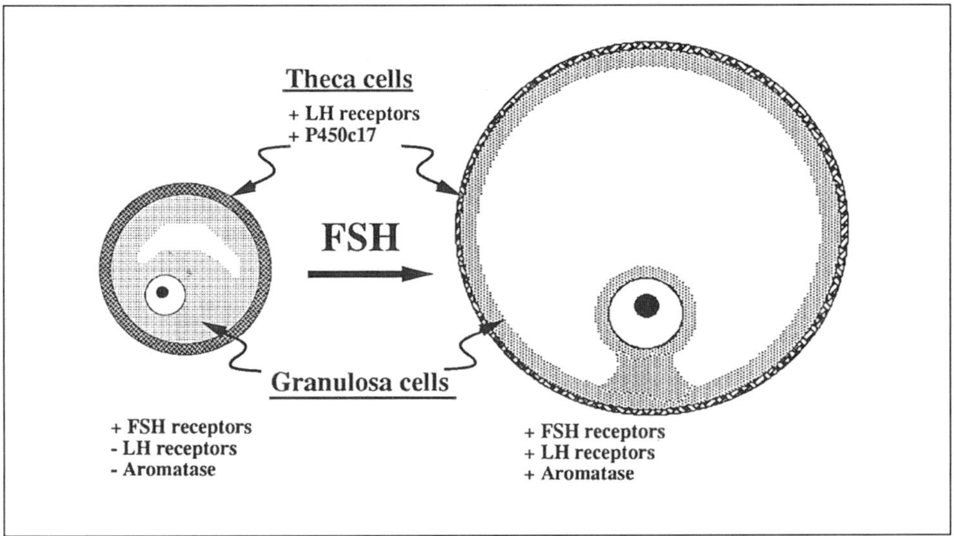

FIGURE 1 - *Characteristics and gonadotropin responsiveness of early antral and preovulatory follicles.*

granulosa cells removed from large follicles demonstrated that the appearance of the LH receptor on granulosa cells is associated with advanced follicle development. The studies of Zeleznik et al.[9] were the first demonstrate that the appearance of LH receptors on granulosa cells was the result of FSH stimulation. It is now generally accepted that FSH is the principal (if not the sole) hormone involved in the initiation of preovulatory follicle development. As a result of FSH stimulation, granulosa cells acquire LH receptors as well as the aromatase enzyme which results in the ability of the follicle to produce estrogen[10].

The essential role of FSH in follicular development in humans has been confirmed by the identification in women of genetic mutations in the FSHß subunit which results in an isolated deficiency of FSH as well as by the identification of inactivating mutations in the gene which encodes for the FSH receptor. Rabin et al.[11] were the first to identify a woman with an isolated deficiency of FSH. This "experiment of nature" had primary amenorrhea, undetectable concentrations of FSH, estrogen concentrations less than 10 pg/ml despite elevated levels of LH and had no antral follicles as assessed by laparoscopy and ovarian biopsy. Ovulation and successful pregnancy occurred in this patient after treatment with FSH[12]. A second such patient with the same clinical manifestations has been identified more recently[13,14]. Interestingly, although unrelated, both subjects shared the same mutation in the FSHß gene that resulted in the production of a truncated FSHß subunit. Additional genetic evidence for the obligatory role of FSH in preovulatory follicle development has been obtained from the identification of inactivating mutations of the FSH receptor in women. This rare disorder is characterized by primary amenorrhea which is associated with the failure of follicles to advance to large antral stages[15]. Interestingly, although patients with inactivating mutations of the FSH receptor do exhibit early stages of follicular development, the number of developing follicles is reported to be less than that seen in women with normal FSH receptors. This raises the possibility that early stages of preantral follicle development may be regulated by FSH, a concept that would appear to be in contrast with the generally accepted view that preantral follicular development may be gonadotropin independent.

LH. As revealed by autoradiographical studies, theca cells of virtually all antral follicles posess LH receptors[5]. Unlike granulosa cells, theca cells express P450c17, the enzyme necessary to convert C21 progestins into C19 androgens, and the capacity of theca cells to produce androgens is governed by LH[7]. As noted previously, granulosa cells of early antral follicles lack LH receptors and are unresponsive to LH. Thus, the theca cells are the principal ovarian cell type regulated by LH during the early stages of preovulatory follicle development. The "two cell - two gonadotropin" model for estrogen synthesis is based upon studies by Falck and others[16,17]. These studies demonstrated that neither granulosa cells nor theca cells alone are capable of producing substantial amounts of estrogen while the combination of these two cell types results in dramatic increases in estrogen secretion. Because theca cells lack the aromatase enzyme necessary to convert androgens to estrogens and granulosa cells lack the P450c17 enzyme which is necessary to produce androgens, the synergistic actions between theca cells and granulosa cells involves theca cell androgen production in response to LH and the stimulation of granulosa cell aromatase by FSH which converts the thecally derived androgens to estrogen. As virtually all antral follicles posess LH receptors and P450c17, the rate limiting stem in estrogen production is the induction of aromatase in granulosa cells by FSH.

Inactivating mutations of the LH receptor have been identified recently in humans. The ovarian phenotype in these individuals is exactly what would have been predicted from the extant knowledge of the effects of LH on the maturing follicle. Thus, women with inactivating mutations of the LH receptor are hypoestrogenic and anovulatory[18]. Interestingly, ovaries in one subject with a nonfunctional LH receptor were reported to be enlarged and polycystic[18].

The likely reason for the ovarian enlargement is that serum FSH concentrations are above normal due to the lack of estrogen mediated negative feedback.

While the role of LH on theca cell function has been well studied, the significance of the FSH-mediated induction of LH receptors on granulosa cells is less appreciated. Undoubtedly, the presence of LH receptors on granulosa cells enables the preovulatory follicle ovulate and luteinize in response to the midcycle LH surge[19]. However, as to be discussed later, the FSH-mediated induction of LH receptors on granulosa cells may also play a paramount role in the process of follicle selection itself.

Follicle selection – current views

Substantial progress has been made in identifying the physiological mechanisms responsible for follicle selection and the transfer of the information gained from experimental animal models into clinical practice. In simple terms, the process of follicle selection must involve a mechanism by which the presence of a maturing follicle inhibits the maturation of other follicles without compromising its own development. Studies in both monkeys[20] and humans[21] have shown that the absolute plasma concentration of FSH is critical for both the initiation of preovulatory follicle development at the beginning of the menstrual cycle as well as for the selection process itself. Figure 2 summarizes the current views on the role of FSH on the initiation of follicle development and follicle selection. During the luteal phase of the menstrual cycle serum concentrations of FSH are maintained below threshold levels and follicular development does not proceed beyond the early antral stages[22]. Upon the regression of the corpus luteum, feedback inhibition of gonadotropin secretion is relieved, FSH secretion increases and plasma concentrations of FSH rise above the threshold necessary to initiate preovulatory follicular development. As a direct consequence of FSH stimulation, aromatase is induced in the granulosa cells of the FSH stimulated follicle and plasma concentrations of estradiol increase. The increase in serum estradiol levels suppresses FSH secretion below threshold levels and the maturation of other lesser mature follicles is curtailed. Experimental evidence for this model was first obtained from subhuman primates and has since been shown to be applicable to humans[21,23].

Thus, follicle selection in humans and subhuman primates involves a process by which the presence of a maturing follicle inhibits the maturation of other less mature follicles by suppressing FSH secretion so that plasma FSH concentrations fall below that necessary to maintain their growth. The final

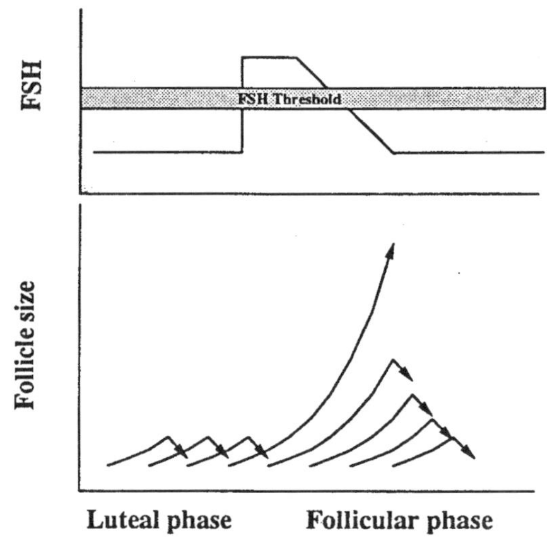

FIGURE 2 - *The role of changes in plasma FSH concnetrations on the initiation of preovulatory follicle development and the selection of a single preovulatory follicle: The threshold theory.*

key question that must be answered to solve the problem of follicle selection is the identification of the cellular mechanisms by which the selected follicle is sparred from its self-imposed reduction in plasma FSH levels – in other words, what allows the maturing follicle to become resistant to the fall in plasma FSH concentrations?

Potential Mechanisms Responsible for the Enhanced Sensitivity of the Maturing Follicle to FSH

The fact that the selected follicle continues to mature in the presence of FSH concentrations which are insufficient to maintain the development of less mature follicles indicates that there must be a specific functional change or changes in the FSH-stimulated follicle that renders it less dependent on FSH than other lesser mature follicles. A number of possible mechanism exist that could explain how the maturing follicle becomes less dependent upon FSH thereby securing its dominance during the mid through late follicular phase of the menstrual cycle. The following section presents a brief description of some of the factors that may influence the responsiveness of follicles to FSH.

Autocrine and paracrine agents

A number of locally produced ovarian factors have been show to synergize with or antagonize the actions of FSH and LH on the developing follicle. The selective production of a positive co-regulator of FSH action or the cessation of the production of a negative co-regulator of FSH action could, in theory, be responsible for the continued maturation of the dominant follicle in the presence of declining FSH concentrations.

While there is ample evidence from *in vitro* studies that many agents have actions on the ovarian follicle, this area of investigation remains limited by a lack of studies conducted *in vivo* to determine the physiological importance of their actions. However, as noted previously, the identification of genetic mutations in FSH and LH receptors has provided conclusive evidence on the roles of FSH and LH in follicular development. In some cases, mutations that affect the production of intraovarian factors may also provide information regarding their importance *in vivo*.

IGF-I. *In vitro* studies with isolated ovarian cells from both rats and humans have shown that IGF I exerts a potent synergistic action upon the effects of FSH and LH. In theca cells, IGF I synergize with LH to promote androgen production[24]. In granulosa cells, IGF I synergizes with FSH to promote the induction of LH receptors and aromatase[24]. In view of the pronounced effects of IGF I on ovarian cellular function and its ability to synergize with FSH to promote the expression of many of the genes that accompany preovulatory follicular development, it is tempting to speculate that this peptide may be involved in protecting the maturing follicle from the progressive fall in FSH concentrations that occurs during the mid through late follicular phase of the menstrual cycle.

Despite the attractiveness of a potential role of IGF I in the process of follicle selection, a clear relationship between IGF I and follicular development in humans has not surfaced. Thus, selective production of IGF I by the preovulatory follicle in humans has not been demonstrated[25], as might be expected if it were to play a role in the selection process. However, the *in vivo* bioactivity of IGF I may be influenced by its sequestration by IGF binding proteins (IGFBP's) such that changes in the concentrations of IGFBP's within the follicle could alter the concentration of "free" IGF I and thereby provide the follicle with increased sensitivity to FSH. While this remains an interesting possibility, comprehensive studies to determine the concentration of biologically active IGF I in the antral fluids of dominant versus non dominant follicles have not been reported.

Perhaps the most significant argument against a role for IGF I *in vivo* comes from another "gene knockout" identified in humans. Laron dwarfs lack the growth hormone receptor hence GH-mediated production of IGF I by the liver does not occur. Women with this defect have ovulatory menstrual cycles and are fertile, despite the absence of IGF I[26]. Moreover, one such subject underwent exogenous gonadotropin therapy for *in vitro* fertilization and responded to a typical regimen (225 IU hMG per day) with elevated estrogen production and the maturation of numerous follicles with oocyte competent of being fertilized[27]. Analysis of follicular fluids from this patient revealed levels of estrogen and progesterone comparable to those of normal women but IGF I concentrations were 1/20th of normal values.

Thus, a critical role for IGF I on follicle selection has yet to be documented. However it is unknown if other factors such as IGF II could be involved in follicular development.

Inhibin/activin system. Conceptually, the intraovarian inhibin/activin system continues to be an attractive candidate for an intraovarian regulatory system. As assesses by in situ hybridization for the subunits of inhibin and activin, the expression of these proteins appears to be developmentally regulated[28]. In the monkey ovary, mRNA for the ßB subunit of inhibin is expressed in granulosa cells of virtually all nonatretic preantral follicles. Because these follicles do not express detectable levels of the α subunit mRNA, it would appear that these follicles are under the tonic control of activin B. In contrast, maturing preovulatory follicles predominantly express mRNAs for the α subunit of inhibin and the ßA subunit suggesting that follicle selection is associated with a switch from the expression of activin B to inhibin A. Inhibin and activin appear to play an important role in the coordination of theca and granulosa cell production of estrogen. As noted previously, the "two cell - two gonadotropin" model for estradiol production involves the stimulation of theca cell androgen production by LH and the induction of aromatase by FSH. Most, if not all antral follicles contain LH receptors and antral fluid androgens are comparable in dominant and non dominant follicles[29]. This would imply that follicles with aromatase must produce more androgens than follicles without aromatase in order to maintain equivalent antral fluid androgen levels. How the theca of the dominant follicle knows that its partner granulosa cells has aromatase could due to activin and inhibin. Activin inhibits LH stimulated androgen production by theca cells while inhibin enhances LH dependent theca androgen production[30]. Thus, in early antral follicles before FSH stimulation and the concomitant induction of aromatase, theca cell LH secretion would be restrained by activin. As the follicle is stimulated by FSH, aromatase is induced which would require increased production of androgens by the theca. The production of inhibin by FSH stimulated follicles would enhance theca cell androgen production and thus provide increased amounts of androgen necessary for aromatization into estradiol.

Estrogen. Based upon studies in rodents that demonstrated a pronounced synergistic effect of estrogen on FSH-mediated granulosa cell function, it has been generally inferred that the rising concentrations of estrogen in the antral fluid of the dominant follicle could impart the granulosa cells of that follicle a greater sensitivity to FSH and thereby provide a cellular mechanism to how the maturing follicle may be spared from the fall in FSH concentrations during the mid through late follicular phase of the menstrual cycle. To date however, this hypothesis is not supported by direct experimental evidence. Thus Koering was unable to demonstrate a stimulatory effect of diethylstilbestrol on either preantral or FSH-stimulated antral follicle development in monkeys[31]. More recently, the demonstration of large multicystic ovaries in women with a genetic defect in aromatase further suggests that estrogens do not play an indispensable role in follicular development[32].

Angiogenesis. The effective concentration of blood borne substances within a tissue compartment is a function of the plasma concentration of the substance and the surface area and permeability of the microvascular capillaries within the tissue that govern the diffusion of the substance from blood into the extracellular fluid that bathes the cells. Morphometric analysis of monkey ovaries demonstrated that the density of capillaries within the theca layer of the dominant follicle was at least 3x greater than that of other smaller follicles. Moreover, this same study demonstrated that the increased capillary density of the dominant follicle was associated with the greater delivery of intravenously administered radiolabeled human chorionic gonadotropin to the dominant follicle when compared with other less mature follicles[33]. It is therefore possible that the angiogenesis that accompanies follicle selection could provide a greater delivery of gonadotropins to the that follicle despite the fact that FSH concentrations are falling.

Recent studies have suggested that vascular endothelial growth factor (VEGF) may be responsible for the angiogenesis that accompanies follicle selection. This protein, a member of the heparin-binding family of growth factors has been shown to promote angiogenesis in both *in vivo* and *in vitro* bioassays[34]. In situ hybridization analysis for VEGF mRNA in the primate ovary revealed that the expression of this mRNA was confined to the mural granulosa cells of the dominant follicle and the corpus luteum[35]. More recent studies have shown that granulosa cells from preovulatory monkey follicles produce immunoreactive VEGF *in vitro* in response to both FSH and LH[36].

Whether the production of VEGF or the angiogenesis that accompanies it is a principal component of the process of follicle selection remains to be demonstrated. The recent identification of specific inhibitors of angiogenesis which are effective *in vivo*[37] may now permit direct analysis of the role of VEGF in the process of follicle selection.

Gonadotropin receptors. A hallmark action of FSH during preovulatory follicular development is the induction of LH receptors on granulosa cells[9]. As shown in Figure 3, granulosa cells from early antral follicles posess FSH receptors and stimulation of the cells by FSH results in the activation of adenylyl cyclase and the production of cAMP. In response to FSH stimulation, granulosa cells acquire LH receptors and, like that the FSH receptor, occupancy of the LH receptor by LH also results in the activation of adenylyl cyclase and the production of cAMP[38]. As would be predicted by the common intracellular cAMP pathway, granulosa cells from FSH stimulated follicles respond similarly to both FSH and LH and moreover, at non-saturating levels of FSH and LH, the responses are additive[39]. The overall significance of these findings is that while granulosa cells from early antral follicles are *only* responsive to FSH, granulosa cells from FSH stimulated follicles are responsive to *either* FSH *or* LH.

In 1984 Zeleznik and Hillier hypothesized that the acquisition of LH receptors on granulosa cells during preovulatory follicle development could consti-

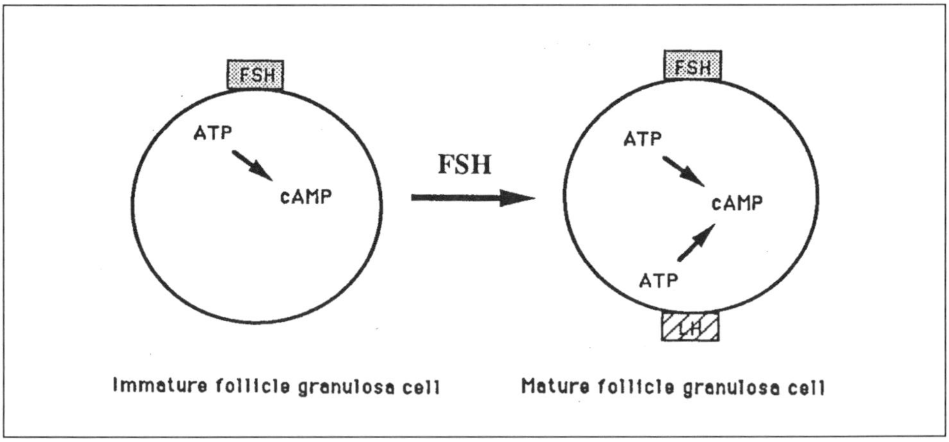

FIGURE 3 - *Hormone effector systems in immature and mature follicles.*

tute a mechanism by which the maturing follicle could be protected from the decline in FSH secretion that occurs during the mid through late follicular phase of the menstrual cycle[40]. The basis for this thesis are the observations that granulosa cells collected from early antral follicles collected at the end of the luteal phase of the human menstrual cycle are responsive to FSH, as assessed by the ability of FSH to induce aromatase activity *in vitro*. However, addition of hCG as a surrogate for LH to these granulosa cells from immature follicles was unable to stimulate aromatase activity. In contrast, aromatase activity of granulosa cells removed from human preovulatory follicles was responsive to the addition of either FSH or LH[29]. Thus, because early antral follicles are responsive to only FSH, a fall in the plasma FSH concentrations would remove the only gonadotropin stimulus capable of sustaining granulosa cell differentiation. In contrast, maturing follicles whose granulosa cells possess LH receptors would be protected from the fall in FSH concentrations because they would be capable of responding to LH as well as FSH. Moreover, although plasma FSH concentrations fall during the mid through late follicular phase of the menstrual cycle, plasma LH concentrations are stable during this time, likely because the sensitivity of FSH to the negative feedback effects of estrogen is greater than that of LH[41,42].

To date, the hypothesizes that the induction of LH receptors is the mechanism by which the selected follicle is protected from the fall in plasma FSH concentrations has been untestable because of a lack of sufficient amounts of purified FSH and LH for use in humans. The recent availability of pure FSH and LH obtained by recombinant DNA technology has now provided the necessary reagents to further explore a role for LH in the process of follicle selection.

As presented in detail elsewhere[43], we tested the hypothesis that the acquisition of LH responsiveness by the maturing follicle contributes to (or is responsible for) the maintenance of the development of the maturing follicle in the presence of declining concentrations of FSH during the mid through late follicular phase of the menstrual cycle. For this purpose twenty-four women with unexplained infertility were treated with a GnRH agonist to interrupt spontaneous gonadotropin secretion. After adequate pituitary desensitization, each woman was treated with recombinant human FSH (Gonal-F, Serono Laboratories, Inc.) at a dosage of 150 or 225 IU/day until one or more follicles reached an average diameter of 14 mm. Thereafter, they were randomized in a double blind manner to one of four treatment groups. Group A subjects discontinued FSH and received saline bi-daily injections for two days. Group B subjects continued to receive FSH for an additional two days. Group C subjects discontinued FSH and received human recombinant LH (LHadi,

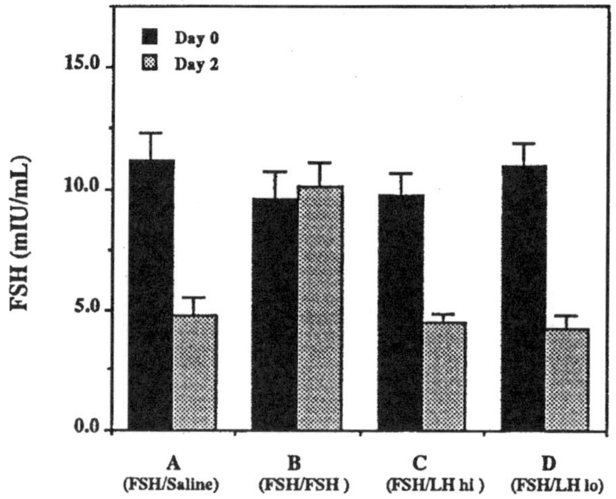

FIGURE 4 - *Mean serum FSH concentration (IU/L) ± SEM of the four treatment groups (A,B,C,D) on the day of randomization (day 0; black bars) and the day of hCG administration (Day 2; gray bars).* Reproduced from reference 43 with permission.

Serono Laboratories, Inc.) at a dosage of 750 IU/d) for two days and Group D subjects discontinued FSH and received recombinant human LH at a dosage of 300 IU/d for two days. Twenty-four hr after the final saline or gonadotropin injection, each subject received 10,000 IU hCG. Serum estrogen concentrations were assessed daily as an index of follicular maturation.

Figure 4 illustrates serum FSH concentrations in the individual treatment groups on the day of randomization (Day 0) and immediately preceding the hCG injections (Day 2). Serum FSH concentrations on the day of randomization (Day 0) were similar in all subjects. As expected, serum FSH concentrations in those subjects that discontinued FSH and received either saline (Group) or LH (Groups C and D) fell while FSH concentrations those subjects who continued to receive FSH (Group B) were maintained at pre-randomization values.

Figure 5 illustrates serum LH concentrations in the four treatment groups. On the day of randomization, all subjects had low concentrations of LH (1-1.5 mIU/ml). Serum LH concentrations in those subjects that received either saline or FSH (Groups A and B) remained at this low level throughout the randomization period. As expected, plasma LH concentrations were elevated in those subjects that received recombinant LH (Groups C and D).

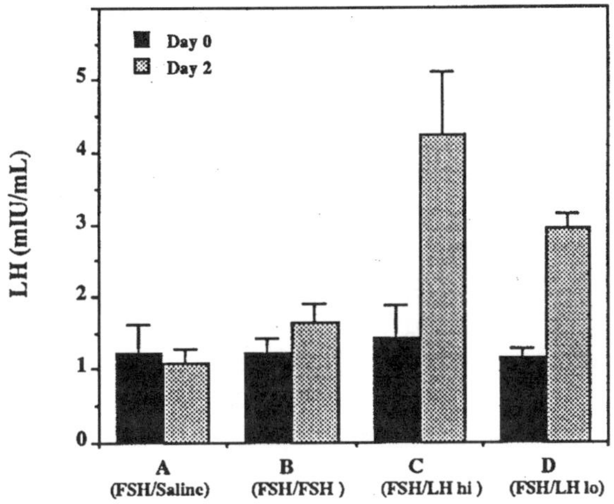

FIGURE 5 - *Mean serum LH concentration (IU/L) ± SEM of the four treatment groups (A,B,C,D) on the day of randomization (Day 0; black bars) and the day of hCG administration (Day 2; gray bars).* Reproduced from reference 43 with permission.

Figure 6 illustrates serum estrogen concentrations in the different treatment groups. In those subjects that received saline during the randomization period (Group A) serum estrogen concentrations rose for one day after the withdrawal of FSH but fell by the second day of randomization. In contrast, in those subjects that continued to receive FSH (Group B) or those who received LH (Groups C and D), serum estrogen concentrations role throughout the entire randomization period. No pregnancies occurred in the saline treated subjects while one pregnancy occurred in each of groups B, C and D.

Implications of the "LH Theory"

The aforementioned observations are consistent with the hypothesis that the maturing follicle may be spared from its self-imposed reduction in serum FSH concentrations by developing the ability to respond to LH, as illustrated in Figure 7. If so, this would indicate that the FSH mediated induction of aromatase concurrent with the induction of LH receptors are the principal mechanisms responsible for the process of follicle selection. The induction of aromatase results in the rise in peripheral levels of estrogen which, as noted earlier, suppress FSH secretion such that plasma concentrations of FSH fall below the threshold that is necessary to stimulate the maturation of other less mature follicles. The concurrent induction of LH receptors provides the maturing follicle with an additional source of tropic support which enables it to continue to mature in the presence of FSH concentrations which are insufficient to support the development of other follicles.

Our current observations would also indicate that, in the absence of adequate gonadotropic support other potential autocrine or paracrine agents are unable to maintain preovulatory follicular development when FSH concentrations decline during the mid through late follicular phase of the menstrual cycle. As all subjects received identical FSH treatment prior to the double-blinded randomization, the intrafollicular milieu of autocrine and paracrine factors in the individual treatment groups should have been similar prior to the randomization. As shown in Figure 6, serum estrogen concentrations in the group of subjects that were randomized to the saline group (Group A) declined following two days while estrogen levels in those subjects that received either FSH (Group B) or LH (Groups C and D) rose throughout the entire period of treatment (Group B, C and D). If factors other than gonadotropins were able to maintain follicular development, we would have expected that serum estrogen concentrations would have continued to rise following

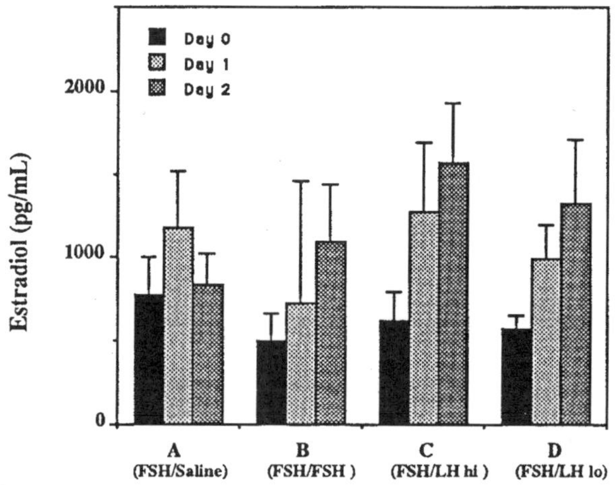

FIGURE 6 - *Results show the mean serum E2 concentrations (pg/ml) ± SEM of the four treatment groups (A,B,C,D) throughout the study period (Days 0, 1 and 2).* Reproduced from reference 43 with permission.

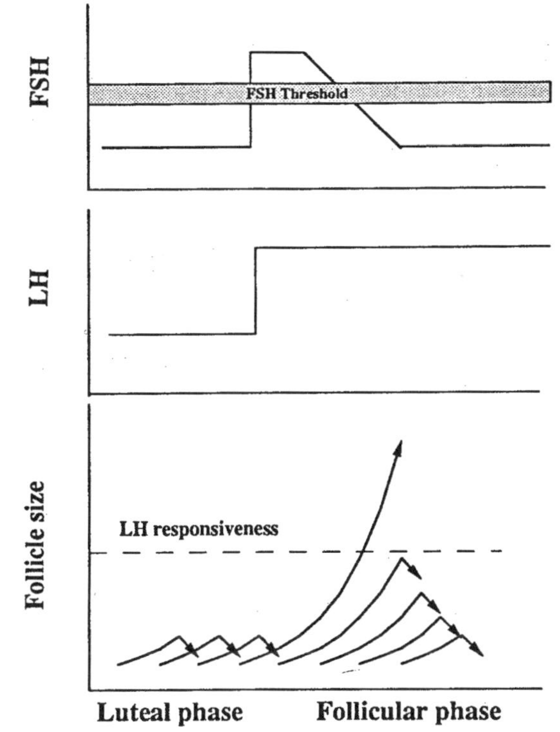

FIGURE 7 - *Proposed role for LH in the process of follicle selection. The acquisition of LH responsivess during FSH-stimulated preovulatory follicular development may provide a mechanism by which the maturing follicle is protected from a fall in plasma FSH concentrations.*

the cessation of FSH treatment, which did not happen.

Finally, these current studies may provide a novel approach for controlled ovarian stimulation in humans. If a specific "cut off point" could be identified below which follicles are unresponsive to LH, it may be possible to develop a sequential FSH/LH stimulation regimen which would be effective in limiting follicular recruitment which could reduce the risk of unplanned ovarian hyperstimulation. Additional studies will be required to determine at which stage of preovulatory follicular development the maturing follicle acquires sufficient LH responsiveness to allow it to escape the fall in serum FSH concentrations.

Acknowledgments

We thank Dr. Louis O'Dea, Ms. Kate Banks and Ms. Marsha Yarkosky from Serono Laboratories, Inc. for providing us with the recombinant FSH and LH and TAP Pharmaceuticals for providing Lupron. The authors research presented in this chapter was supported in part by NIH grants HD 08610 and HD 12014.

References

1. Greep R.O., Van Dyke H.B., Chow B.F.: Gonadotropins of the swine pituitary: various biological effects of purified thylakentrin (FSH) and pure metakentrin (ICSH). *Endocrinology*, 30:635-649, 1942.
2. Knobil E., Kostyo J.L., Greep R.O.: Production of ovulation in the hypophysectomized rhesus monkey. *Endocrinology*, 65:487-493, 1959.
3. Gemzell C.: Induction of ovulation with human gonadotropins. *Rec. Prog. Hormone Res.*, 21:179-204, 1965.
4. vanWagenen G.: Induction of ovulation in *Macaca mulatta*. *Fertil. Steril.*, 19: 15-29, 1968.
5. Midgley A.R. Jr.: Autoradiographic analysis of gonadotropin binding to rat ovarian tissue sections. *Adv. Exp. Biol. Med.*, 36:365-378, 1973.
6. Channing C.P.: Influences of the *in vivo* and *in vitro* hormonal environment upon luteinization of granulosa cells in tissue culture. *Rec. Prog. Hormone Res.*, 26:589-622, 1970.
7. Erickson G.F., Magoffin D.A., Dyer C.A., Hofeditz C.: The ovarian androgen producing cells: a review of structure/function relationships. *Endocrine Rev.*, 6:371-399, 1985.
8. Channing C.P., Kammerman S.: Characteristics of gonadotropin receptors on granulosa cells during folicular maturation. *Endocrinology*, 92:531-540, 1973.
9. Zeleznik A.J., Midgley A.R. Jr., Reichert L.E. Jr.: Granulosa cell matauration in the rat: increased binding of human chorionic gonadotropin following treatment with follicle stimulating hormone *in vivo*. *Endocrinology*, 95:818-825, 1974.
10. Erickson G.F., Hsueh A.J.W.: Stimulation of aromatase activity by follicle stimulating hormone in rat granulosa cells *in vivo* and *in vitro*. *Endocrinology*, 102:1275-1283, 1978.
11. Rabin D., Spitz I., Bercovici B., Bell J., Laufer A., Benvieniste R., Polishuk W.: Isolated deficiency of follicle stimulating hormone. *New England J. Med.*, 287:1313-1317, 1972.
12. Rabinowicz D., Benveniste R., Lindner J., Lorber D., Daniell J.: Isolated

follicle stimulating hormone deficiency revisited. *New England J. Med.*, 300: 126-128, 1979.
13. Matthews C.H., Borgato S., Beck-Peccoz P., Adams M., Tone Y., Gambino G., Casagrande S., Tedeschini G., Benedetti A., Chatterjee V.K.: Primary amenorrhea due to a mutation in the beta-subunit of folicle stimulating hormone. *Nature Genetics*, 5:83-86, 1993.
14. Matthews C.H., Chatterjee V.K.: Isolated deficiency of follicle stimulating hormone revisited. *New England J. Med.*, 337:642, 1997.
15. Aittomaki K., Herva R., Stenman U.H., Juntunen K., Ylostalo P., Hovatta O., de la Chapelle A.: Clinical features of primary ovarian failure caused by a point mutation in the follicle stimulating hormone receptor gene. *J. Clin. Endocrinol. Metab.*, 81:3722-3726, 1996.
16. Falck B.: Site of production of estrogen in rat ovary as studied by micro-transplants. *Acta Physiol. Scand. Suppl.*, 163 47:1-101, 1959.
17. Zeleznik A.J., Hillier S.G.: The ovary: endocrine function. In: Hillier S.G., Kitchener H.C., Neilson J.P., *Scientific Essentials of Reproductive Medicine.* W.B. Saunders Co. Ltd. London, pp. 133-146.
18. Toledo S.P., Brunner H.G., Kraaij R., Post M., Dahia P.L., Hayashida C.Y., Kremer H., Themmen A.P.: An inactivating mutation of the luteinizing hormone receptor causes amenorrhea in a 46,XX female. *J. Clin. Endocrinol. Metab.*, 81:3850-3854, 1996.
19. Zeleznik A.J., Keyes P.L., Menon K.M.J., Midgley A.R. Jr., Reichert L.E. Jr.: Development-dependent responses of ovarian follicles to FSH and hCG. *Am. J. Physiol.*, 233:E229-234, 1977.
20. Zeleznik A.J., Kubik C.J.: Ovarian responses in macaques to pulsatile infusion of follicle stimulating hormone and luteinizing hormone: increased sensitivity of the maturing follicle to FSH. *Endocrinology*, 119:2025-2032, 1986.
21. Fauser B.C.J., Van Heusden A.M.: Manipulation of human ovarian function: physiolgical concepts and clinical consequences. *Endocrine Rev.*, 18:71-106, 1997.
22. Zeleznik A.J., Wildt L., Schuler H.M.: Characterization of ovarian folliculogenesis during the luteal phase of the menstrual cycle in rhesus monkeys using [3H] thymidine autoradiography. *Endocrinology*, 107:982-988, 1980.
23. Taymor M.L.: The regulation of follicle growth: some clinical implications in reproductive endocrinology. *Fertil. Steril.*, 65:235-247, 1996.
24. Bergh C., Carlsson B., Olsson J.-H., Selleskog U., Hillensjo T.: Regulation of androgen production by cultured human thecal cells by insulin-like growth factor and insulin. *Fertil. Steril.*, 59:323-330, 1993.
25. Hernandez E.R., Hurwitz A., Vera A., Pellicer A., Adashi E., LeRoith D.,

Roberts C.T. Jr.: Expression of the genes encoding the insulin-like growth factors and their receptors in the human ovary. *J. Clin. Endocrinol. Metab.*, 74: 419-425, 1992.

26. Laron Z.: Laron syndrome: from description to therapy. *Endocrinologist*, 3:21-28, 1993.
27. Dor J., Ben-Shlomo I., Lunenfeld B., Pariente C., Levran D., Karasik A., Seppälä M., Masiach S.: Insulin-like growth factor-I (IGF-I) may not be essential for ovarian follicular development: evidence from IGF deficiency. *J. Clin. Endocrinol. Metab.*, 74:539-542, 1992.
28. Schwall R.H., Mason A.J., Wilcox J.N., Bassett S.G., Zeleznik A.J.: Localization of inhibin/activin subunit mRNAs within the primate ovary. *Mol. Endocrinol.*, 4:75-79, 1990.
29. Hillier S.G., Reichert L.E. Jr., van Hall E.V.: Control of preovulatory follicular estrogen biosynthesis in the human ovary. *J. Clin. Endocrinol. Metab.*, 52:847-856, 1981.
30. Hillier S.G.: Paracrine control of follicular estrogen synthesis. *Sem. Reprod. Endocrinol.*, 4:332-340, 1991.
31. Koering M.J.: Follicular maturation and atresia: morphological correlates. In: R. Stouffer, R. Brenner and C. Phoenix (eds), *The Primate Ovary*, pp. 3-23., Plenum Press, New York, 1987.
32. Morishima A., Grumbach M.M., Simpson E.R., Fisher C., Qin K.: Aromatase deficiency in male and female siblings caused by a novel mutation and the physiological role of estrogens. *J. Clin. Endocrinol. Metab.*, 80:3689-3698, 1995.
33. Zeleznik A.J., Schuler H.M., Reichert L.E. Jr.: Gonadotropin-binding sites in the rhesus monkey ovary: role of the vasculature in the selective distribution of human chorionic gonadotropin to the preovulatory follicle. *Endocrinology*, 109:356-362, 1981.
34. Ferrara N., Houck K., Jakeman L., Leung D.W.: Molecular and biological properties of the vascular endothelial growth factor family of proteins. *Endocrine Rev.*, 13:18-32, 1992.
35. Ravindranath N., Little-Ihrig L.L., Phillips H.S., Ferrara N., Zeleznik A.J.: Vascular endothelial growth factor messenger ribonucleic acid expression in the primate ovary. *Endocrinology*, 131:254-260, 1992.
36. Christensen L.K., Stouffer R.L.: Follicle stimulating hormone and luteinizing hormone/chorionic gonadotropin stimulation of vascular endothelial growth factor production my macaque granulosa cells from pre- and periovulatory follicles. *J. Clin. Endocrinol. Metab.*, 82:2135-2142, 1997.
37. Folkman J.: Is tissue mass regulated by vascular endothelial cells? Prostate as the first evidence. *Endocrinology*, 139:441-442, 1998.

38. Goff A.K., Armstrong D.T.: Stimulatory actions of gonadotropins and prostaglandins on adenosine-3',5'-monophosphate production by isolated rat granulosa cells. *Endocrinology*, 101:1461-1469.
39. Kolena J., Channing C.P.: Stimulatory effects of LH, FSH and prostaglandins upon cyclic 3',5'-AMP levels in porcine granulosa cells. *Endocrinology*, 90:1543-1550.
40. Zeleznik A.J., Hillier S.G.: The role of gonadotropins in the selection of the preovulatory follicle. *Clin. Obstet. Gynecol.*, 27:927-940, 1984.
41. Saketos M., Sharma N., Adel T., Raghuwanshi M., Santoro N.: Time-resolved immunoflorimetric assay and specimen storage conditions for measuring urinary gonadotropins. *Clin. Chem.*, 40:749-753, 1994.
42. Marshall J.C., Case G.D., Valk T.W., Corley K.P., Sauder S.E., Kelch R.P.: Selective inhibition of follicle stimulating hormone secretion by estradiol. Mechanisms for modulation of gonadotropin responses to low dose pulses of gonadotropin releasing hormone. *J. Clin. Invest.*, 71:248-256, 1983.
43. Sullivan M.W., Stewart-Aikers A., Krasnow J.S., Berga S.L., Zeleznik A.J.: Ovarian responses in women to recombinant follicle stimulating hormone and luteinizing hormone: a role for LH in the final stages of follicular matauration. *J. Clin. Endocrtinol. Metab.*, 84:228-232, 1999.

The Role of Luteinizing Hormone
in Folliculogenesis
and Ovulation Induction,, pp. 21-36
Editor M. Filicori

Specific Roles of Luteinizing Hormone (LH) and Follicle-stimulating Hormone (FSH) in Folliculogenesis and Ovulation

M.B. Zelinski-Wooten, A.M. Weston, D.P. Wolf and R.L. Stouffer

Oregon Regional Primate Research Center, Beaverton, OR (United States of America)

Abstract. *During in vitro fertilization (IVF) cycles, typically FSH and LH are used to induce follicular growth followed by a bolus of human chorionic gonadotropin (hCG) to promote periovulatory events. Although both FSH and LH are required for normal follicular steroidogenesis, the role for LH in follicular growth and oocyte development is unclear. The efficacy of FSH as an alternative to LH/hCG for the initiation of periovulatory events in primate follicles is also unknown. To address these issues, rhesus monkeys received (1) a 90-day exposure to a GnRH antagonist, followed by recombinant (r)-hFSH alone and with r-hLH (1:1, Ares Serono) to promote multiple follicular development and a standard ovulatory dose of urinary hCG (1000 IU); and (2) r-hFSH alone for follicular development followed by a bolus of r-hFSH (2500 IU, Ares Serono) or r-hCG (1000 IU; Ares Serono). A longer interval of r-hFSH exposure (12 ± 1 days) than r-hFSH + r-hLH (9 ± 0.2 days) was required for equivalent, multiple follicular growth. Serum estradiol (E) levels were 4-fold lower with r-hFSH alone versus r-hFSH + r-hLH. After the hCG bolus, more oocytes completed meiosis to metaphase II (51 vs. 12%) and fertilized (89 vs. 52%) in the r-hFSH versus r-hFSH + r-hLH group, respectively. However, a significant decrease in cryosurvival (56 vs. 78%) and rate of in vitro development to hatched blastocyst (10 vs. 12 days) was observed in embryos from r-hFSH vs r-hFSH + r-hLH. Pregnancies resulted from oviductal transfers in both groups. A midcycle bolus of r-hFSH was equivalent to r-hCG for the reinitiation of oocyte meiosis (89 vs. 88%) and fertilization (47 ± 19 vs. 50 ± 7%). Likewise, indices of early granulosa cell luteinization, acute progesterone (P) production in vitro and expression of P receptors, were similar between groups. Thus, a regimen of FSH alone which activates the growth of antral follicles as well as meiotically- and developmentally-competent oocytes, can be combined with a bolus of FSH as an ovulatory stimulus which promotes oocyte maturation, fertilization and early events in follicular luteinization. However, exposure to LH during the preovulatory interval of spontaneous ovarian cycles may a) insure adequate steroidogenesis to support E-mediated effects on target tissues, i.e. the endometrium; and b) enhance embryo viability and the rate of blastocyst* *development. The surges of FSH and LH that occur spontaneously at midcycle may be redundant signals to insure that early periovulatory events occur. Whether FSH can substitute for LH/hCG in primates to evoke follicular rupture and oocyte release, as in rodent models, remains to be tested. Follicular stimulation/ovulation induction regimens composed solely of FSH offer potential clinical utility for reducing ovarian hyperstimulation syndrome, improving fertility in patients with polycystic ovarian syndrome, and reducing infertility in LH-resistant patients.*

Key Words. Embryonic development, follicular stimulation, in vitro fertilization, oocyte maturation, recombinant FSH, recombinant LH.

Introduction

In the natural ovarian cycle, the normal steroidogenic function of the maturing follicle depends upon two pituitary gonadotropins, follicle-stimulating hormone (FSH) and luteinizing hormone (LH). According to the two-cell, two gonadotropin model[1], low levels of LH during the follicular phase act on theca cells to elicit androgen synthesis, which then serves as a substrate for estrogen production by granulosa cells in response to FSH. While this model is valid for steroid production by the primate follicle, the role for LH in supporting growth of the antral follicle, maturation of its enclosed oocyte as well as subsequent fertilization and embryo quality is unclear. The recent availability of recombinant human FSH (r-hFSH) and LH (r-hLH) preparations[2,3] which are devoid of contamination with other gonadotropins has facilitated unequivocal testing of the hypothesis that FSH, in the absence of LH, can promote the growth and function of the antral follicle in primates.

The gonadotropin surge at midcycle in women[4] and non-human primates[5] is characterized by a rise in circulating levels of both FSH as well as LH. Nonetheless, the physiologic events occurring the in the ovulatory follicle, i.e., resumption of oocyte meiosis, luteinization of the follicle wall and ovulation, are attributed generally to LH. Although early studies in laboratory animals suggested a role for FSH in ovulation[6-8], the results were questioned due to residual LH contamination in the FSH preparations used. Recent data emerging from the use of recombinant FSH alone as a midcycle stimulus in rodents confirmed follicle rupture in the absence of a LH surge[9-12]. Similar studies using a bolus of r-hFSH or r-hCG are needed to examine and compare the ability of each gonadotropin to induce periovulatory events in the primate follicle.

Therefore, prospective studies were performed during in vitro fertilization (IVF)-related cycles in rhesus monkeys, in collaboration with Ares Advanced

Technology, Inc., to evaluate the efficacy of r-hFSH alone to (a) promote folliculo- and gametogenic events following 90 days of gonadotropin-releasing hormone (GnRH) antagonist treatment which reduced endogenous gondotropin levels to baseline; and (b) induce periovulatory events when administered as a bolus at midcycle in comparison to a standard ovulatory bolus of human chorionic gonadotropin (hCG).

Methods

Follicular Stimulation with FSH Alone, or FSH + LH. Rhesus monkeys were "medically hypophysectomized" via treatment with the GnRH antagonist, Antide (Laboratoires Serono SA, Aubonne Switzerland; 0.5 mg/kg body weight sc daily) for 90 days prior to and during the IVF cycle[13]. According to the hypothesis of Gougeon[14], follicle growth from the small preantral to the preovulatory stage requires 80-90 days in women. Chronic Antide treatment during the 90-day interval should expose every follicle to a gonadotropin-deficient milieu throughout its growth phase.

To stimulate the growth of multiple follicle development, animals received twice daily injections of either r-hFSH (30 IU, Gonal-F, Laboratoires Serono SA, Aubonne Switzerland) or r-hFSH + r-hLH (30 IU each, Laboratoires Serono SA)[13]. When at least 6 preovulatory follicles ≈ 4 mm diameter were observed by ultrasonography, an ovulatory bolus of urinary (u)-hCG (1000 IU Profasi, Serono Laboratories Inc., Norwell, MA, USA) was given the next day. Follicles were aspirated from anesthetized monkeys 27 h post-hCG injection.

Levels of bioactive LH and FSH, as well as estradiol and progesterone were measured in serum samples obtained from the initiation of Antide treatment through the end of the IVF cycle. Nuclear maturity of oocytes obtained from follicular aspirates was identified after brief exposure to hyaluronidase, classified as germinal vesicle (GV), metaphase I (MI; no GV and no polar body), metaphase II (MII; no GV and one polar body), and inseminated in vitro as previously described[15]. Fertilized oocytes that underwent early cleavage in vitro were cryopreserved[15]. Procedures for embryo co-culture, evaluation and transfer are described in detail By Weston *et al.*[16]. Briefly, embryos were thawed and placed in co-culture with Buffalo rat liver (BRL) cells (CRL 1442, American Type Culture Collection, Rockville, MD, USA) in modified CMRL-1066 media (Gibco, Grand Island, NY, USA) containing 10% fetal bovine serum. Embryo stages were evaluated daily and a differential fluorescent nuclear stain was used to determine the number of inner cell mass and trophectoderm cells in all hatched blastocysts[16]. Additional cryopreserved-thawed embryos were transferred (two embryos per transfer) to the oviduct of recipient females during the early luteal phase of spontaneous menstrual cycles[16]. Embryo viability was examined by ultrasonography, and implantation was confirmed by measuring serum levels of estradiol, progesterone and bioactive LH/macaque CG through day 32 of pregnancy.

Administration of a Midcycle Bolus of r-hFSH or r-hCG. The protocol for stimulation of multiple follicular development is described in detail by Zelinski-Wooten *et al.*[17,18]. To prevent an endogenous LH surge, rhesus monkeys received Antide daily beginning at midluteal phase of a spontaneous menstrual cycle through the day of the ovulatory stimulus. After 7 days of Antide treatment, animals were given r-hFSH (Gonal-F, 30 IU, twice daily, im) until at least 6 preovulatory follicles were observed by ultrasonography as described above. The next day, monkeys received a single im injection of either 1000 IU r-hCG (Laboratoires Serono SA) or 2500 IU r-hFSH (Laboratoires Serono SA). Follicles were aspirated from anesthetized monkeys 27 h after the midcycle bolus injection. Circulating levels of estradiol and progesterone throughout the IVF cycle were determined by radioimmunoassay. Bioactive LH/CG and immunoactive FSH levels were measured at intervals for up to 72 h after the hCG or FSH bolus.

Oocyte maturation and IVF were evaluated as described above[17,18]. Granulosa cells were isolated from the pooled follicular aspirates, purified and cultured in Ham's F10 mediua (Gibco, Grand Island, NY, USA) containing 10% amenorrheic monkey serum, in the absence (basal) or presence of highly purified u-hCG (100 ng/ml CR123, The National Hormone and Pituitary Distribution Program, NIDDK, NIH, USA;[17,18]). Progesterone production in vitro was determined in media collected after 24 h of culture. Granulosa cells were also plated on chamber slides, frozen until detection of progesterone receptors by indirect immunocytochemistry[19]. The percentage of nuclei staining specifically for progesterone receptors was determined by a random count of 500 nuclei.

Results

Folliculo- and Gametogenic Performance: FSH Alone versus FSH + LH. Circulating levels of bioactive LH and FSH decreased relative to pretreatment levels within two days of GnRH antagonist treatment, and remained suppressed throughout the remainder of the 90-day interval. By 30-45 days post-Antide, all animals displayed gonadotropin levels typical of those observed in surgically hypophysectomized female monkeys (≤ 2.5 ng LH/ml; ± 75 ng FSH/ml). Pulsatile LH secretion was absent on day 90 of Antide

TABLE 1 - *Comparison of follicular and oocyte characteristics between monkeys treated with r-hFSH alone or r-hFSH + r-hLH (1:1) for ovarian stimulation.*

	r-hFSH	*r-hFSH + r-hLH*
Interval (days) to achieve 6 follicles ≥ 4 mm diameter	12 ± 1	9 ± 0.2
Serum estradiol levels (pg/ml) on the day prior to hCG bolus	210 ± 30*	700 ± 310
No. large antral follicles/animal on the day of hCG	24 ± 1	24 ± 2
No. oocytes collected/animal 27 h post-hCG	30 ± 10	25 ± 5
Percentage of MI oocytes at collection	35*	70
Percentage of MII oocytes at collection	51*	12
Overall fertilization rate (%)	89 ± 5*	52 ±11

See text and references 13 and 16 for details.
Values represent mean ± SEM; * $P < 0.05$ between r-hFSH alone or with r-hLH.

treatment. Both estradiol and progesterone levels remained at baseline through the 90-day interval of Antide administration. Thus, the chronic Antide regimen suppressed endogenous gonadotropin secretion sufficiently to examine the relative roles of FSH alone or in combination with LH to promote follicle/oocyte growth and maturation in the primate ovary.

Table 1 summarizes follicular and oocyte performance in monkeys receiving r-hFSH alone versus r-hFSH + r-hLH during chronic Antide treatment. The interval required to achieve the predetermined level of follicular growth prior to administration of the hCG bolus was longer (12 days) in animals treated with r-hFSH relative to those that received r-hFSH + r-hLH (9 days). The patterns and levels of serum estradiol differed between groups; levels during the first 5 days of r-hFSH treatment did not rise and subsequently reached values that were 4-5 fold less than those in the r-hFSH + r-hLH group prior to hCG injection[11]. However, the numbers and size distribution of large follicles as well as the number of oocytes collected did not differ between groups.

When follicle development was stimulated with r-hFSH alone, a greater proportion of oocytes continued to mature to the MII stage relative to the r-hFSH + r-hLH group. In addition, the overall fertilization rate for mature oocytes from the r-hFSH group (89%) was superior to that of the r-hFSH + r-hLH group (52%).

TABLE 2 - *Comparison of embryonic development in vitro and in vivo in cryopreserved/thawed embryos derived from rhesus monkeys treated with r-hFSH alone or r-hFSH + r-hLH during follicular stimulation.*

	r-hFSH	*r-hFSH + r-hLH*
Viability post-thaw (% of embryos)	56*	78
Viable embryos (% of total) reaching:		
morula	64	62
blastocyst	36	41
expanded blastocyst	36	31
hatched blastocyst	28	31
Interval (days) required to reach hatched blastocyst in vitro	12 ± 0.4*	10 ± 0.2
No. of cells (% comprising inner cell mass) in hatched blastocysts	569 ± 84 (31)	429 ± 32 (25)
No. pregnancies/no. embryo transfers	1/8	2/3

Adapted from reference 16
Values represent mean ± SEM; *P < 0.05 between r-hFSH alone or r-hFSH + r-hLH.

In contrast, the viability of thawed embryos (i.e. those that did not lyse or fragment and reached the 8-cell stage by day 3 of culture) was greater following follicular stimulation with r-hFSH + r-hLH (Table 2). Although there were no differences in the developmental efficiency of embryos between the groups, the rate of development in vitro was slower from the expanded to the hatched blastocyst stages when embryos were derived from the r-hFSH alone group relative to the r-hFSH + r-hLH group. There were no differences in the total cell number per embryo or the number of cells comprising the inner cell mass in hatched blastocysts of both groups (Table 2).

Two of three animals receiving two embryos derived from r-hFSH + r-hLH treatment became pregnant, had normal gestation lengths and delivered healthy offspring. Corpus luteum rescue, defined as the day that serum LH/CG first rose above baseline, was evident on day 12-13 of the luteal phase and was associated with an increase in circulating progesterone levels[16]. In contrast, only one of eight animals receiving embryos derived from the r-hFSH group became pregnant. Corpus luteum rescue was delayed to day 16, and rising CG levels were not correlated with increasing progesterone levels. However, a twin pregnancy of normal duration resulted in vaginal delivery of a live normal female and Cesarean section of a normal male that died during maternal dystocia[16].

TABLE 3 - *Comparison of the efficacy of u- or r-hCG (1000 IU) versus r-hFSH (2500 IU) as an ovulatory stimulus for periovulatory events and corpus luteum function in rhesus monkeys during IVF-related cycles.*

	u-hCG	*r-hCG*	*r-hFSH*
Oocytes			
No. recovered/animal	29 ± 7	28 ± 8	27 ± 9
MI (%)	61*	44	36
MII (%)	28*	44	53
Overall fertilization rate (%)	50 ± 17	50 ± 18	47 ± 19
Granulosa Cells			
Basal progesterone production (ng/ml) in vitro over 24 h	620 ± 186	530 ± 185	958 ± 464
Progesterone receptor, % positive cells	76 ± 8	67 ± 9	76 ± 5
VEGF production (pg/ml)	Not determined	799 ± 374	675 ± 231
Corpus Luteum			
Serum progesterone levels (ng/ml) on day 6 post-injection	19 ± 12	22 ± 6	6 ± 3*
Luteal phase length (days)	12 ± 1	11 ± 0.2	10 ± 0.2

Derived from references 17 (for u-hCG), 18 (for r-hCG and r-hFSH) and 20 (for VEGF production).
Data represent mean ± SEM; *P <0.05 between groups (ovulatory stimulus) within row.

Induction of Periovulatory Events: hCG versus FSH. Following the bolus injection of r-hCG, bioactive CG levels increased above baseline (1-3 ng/ml) within 30 min. Peak levels of bioactive CG (1200 ng/ml) were sustained for 8-12 h, and "surge levels", i.e. those typical of the midcycle LH surge during a spontaneous menstrual cycle (≥ 100 ng/ml), were evident for > 48 h post-injection. Baseline levels of immunoreactive FSH were 12 mIU/ml prior to the bolus injection of r-hFSH, increased markedly within 30 min post-injection, and were sustained at peak levels (1800 mIU/ml) for 8 h. High FSH levels (> 100 mIU/ml) were still evident for 48 h. Bioactive LH levels remained unchanged throughout the 72 h sampling interval after administration of the r-hFSH bolus[18].

The characteristics of mutiple follicular development including the patterns and levels of circulating estradiol during the interval of follicular stimulation, the total numbers and size distribution of follicles on the day of the ovulatory stimulus, and the number of oocytes collected at follicle aspiration were similar between animals receiving a bolus of r-hCG or r-hFSH at midcycle[18]. Table 3 summarizes oocyte characteristics as well as indices of granulosa cell luteinization and corpus luteum function after administration of 1000 IU r-hCG and 2500 IU r-hFSH. Data from animals receiving 1000 IU urinary hCG[17] are also included for comparative purposes. Reinitation of oocyte meiosis was observed in 88-89% of the total cohort aspirated 27 h after the ovulatory stimulus in all treatment groups, with comparable fertilization rates achieved in vitro. Likewise, basal and hCG-stimulated progesterone production over 24 h by granulosa cells in vitro and the specific expression of progesterone receptors in granulosa cell nuclei at the time of aspiration did not differ among groups[18].

The production of vascular endothelial growth factor (VEGF), proposed to mediate neovascularization of the developing corpus luteum, by granulosa cells in vitro was also equivalent after r-hCG or r-hFSH as the ovulatory stimulus[20]. Following a bolus of 1000 IU u- or r-hCG, serum progesterone levels increased within 24 h, peaked 4-6 days after hCG injection, and then declined to baseline within 5 days. Although peak concentrations of progesterone following the r-hFSH bolus were similar relative to the hCG, levels were declining by day 4 post-FSH injection and were less than in hCG-treated animals thereafter until reaching baseline[18]. In all cases, the length of the luteal phase did not differ among groups.

Discussion

Can Normal Folliculo- and Gametogenesis Occur under the Influence of FSH in the Absence of LH? These studies provide novel data comparing the efficacy of r-hFSH alone and in combination with r-hLH to restore folliculogenesis in primates following chronic gonadotropin suppression with a GnRH antagonist. Since similar numbers and sizes of large antral follicles developed during r-hFSH stimulation, LH circulating at concentrations greater than the minimal bioactivity typical of hypophysectomized macaques is not required for follicular growth. Our data in nonhuman primates support those of earlier studies in using urinary gonadotropins[21-23] as well as recent demonstrations that antral follicle growth can proceed with r-hFSH alone in hypogonadotropic women[24,25] and macaques[26]. The longer interval of r-hFSH treatment required to attain follicular development prior to administration of the ovulatory hCG stimulus may be related to the dose of FSH used[25]. Alternatively, FSH may synergize with LH to promote follicle growth via production of locally produced growth factors[27,28]. The greater estradiol levels achieved during follicular stimulation with r-hFSH + r-hLH relative to those of r-hFSH alone in our study support the “two-cell, two gonadotropin” concept of follicular steroidogenesis. Interestingly, when macaques were treated with r-hFSH alone, levels of estradiol typical of those produced by a single preovulatory follicle during a natural menstrual cycle were noted. Estradiol synthesis in the absence of LH is somewhat paradoxical if the "two-cell, two gonadotropin" concept is true. It is unknown whether adrenal androgens serve as substrates for aromatization to estrogen, or the very low level of LH bioactivity is sufficient to support a degree of androgen production by theca cells. The latter possibility is supported by studies in hypophysectomzied rats wherein r-hFSH administration in vivo upregulates thecal androgen synthesis via the production of a granulosa-derived paracrine factor when r-hLH is administered in doses that are nondetectable in the circulation[29]. Estradiol synthesis in hypogonadotropic hypogonadal women is very low during treatment with r-hFSH alone[24,25,30], suggesting a greater degree of LH deprivation than we may have observed in macaques during chronic Antide treatment. Restoration of normal estradiol synthesis in hypogonadotropic hypogonadal women required at least half as much r-hLH relative to a constant dose of r-hFSH[30]. In contrast, increasing doses of r-hFSH resulted in substantial levels of circulating estradiol ($\approx$ 225 pg/ml) in a patient with a similar gonadotropin deficiency[31]. Nonetheless, in both gonadotropin-suppressed macaques[13,26] and women[24,25,30,31] the development of multiple antral follicles occurred with r-hFSH alone. This observation also adds to the mounting evidence that increasing estradiol levels are not required for follicular development and granulosa cell proliferation in primates[32]. The extent to which follicular estradiol synthesis occurs may be correlated with the number of preovulatory follicles that develop in response to FSH alone or a "threshold" level of LH that may be higher in some cases, or extremely low (absent?) in hypogonadotropic hypogonadal women[28]. Whether estradiol production following r-hFSH treatment is sufficient to support estradiol-mediated effects on target tissues such as the uterine endometrium is not known.

Following the ovulatory hCG stimulus, oocyte nuclear maturation and fertilizability were consistently greater when follicle development occurred with r-hFSH alone relative to r-hFSH + r-hLH (1:1). Chronic Antide administration combined with subsequent r-hFSH treatment may provide more synchronous development and maturation of a follicular cohort resulting in improved oocyte performance relative to r-hFSH + r-hLH. Alternatively, the presence of equal amounts of FSH and LH during antral follicular development may be deleterious to oocyte meiotic maturation and fertilization. The threshold of LH or ratio of FSH:LH that result in suboptimal oocyte performance is not known. Conversely, fertilization of oocytes derived from follicles stimulated with r-hFSH alone in a hypogonadotropic hypogonadal woman was lower than that observed in a previous stimulation cycle with human menopausal gonadotropin[31], suggesting that some level of LH exposure during the preovulatory period may be necessary for normal gametogenic functions.

The developmental potential of IVF-produced embryos from both treatment groups was similar with respect to the ability of developing embryos to cleave and produce blastocysts with a definitive inner cell mass during in vitro culture. However, two notable differences were also observed. First, embryos derived from r-hFSH treatment alone exhibited reduced viability after thawing. Enhanced cryosurvival of early cleavage stage embryos may be related to as yet undiscovered LH-dependent cytoplasmic or membrane functions that reduce cryodamage. Second, development from the morula to blastocyst stage was slower in embryos derived from r-hFSH treatment relative to r-hFSH + r-hLH. Differences in the follicular milieu during the pre- or periovulatory period may affect post-fertilization development. Inclusion of LH in the follicular stimulation protocol enhanced follicular production of estradiol and presumably androgens, that may regulate oocyte maturation necessary for post-fertilization events in primates[16,32]. However, inclusion of estradiol treatment concomitant with r-hFSH stimulation did not affect fertilization in a hypogonadotropic hypogonadal woman[31] supporting earlier reports that estradiol is not an absolute requirement for gametogenesis in women[32]. The production of local non-steroidal factors that ultimately improve the rate of embryo development may occur via synergistic actions of LH with FSH[16]. The data also suggest that the shorter interval of follicular growth in the r-hFSH + r-hLH group may also contribute to the more rapid development of embryos relative to those derived from r-hFSH alone.

The small number of embryo transfers performed in macaques precludes definitive conclusions regarding the necessity for LH during antral follicular development to contribute to normal embryonic development in vivo. The lower incidence of implantation after transfer of r-hFSH-derived embryos corresponded to their slower developmental rate in vitro, as well as to a delay in the rescue of the corpus luteum by macaque CG in vivo. Although the use of r-hFSH alone for ovarian stimulation in women has resulted in live births (for review,[16,33]), it cannot be ascertained from these case reports whether this regimen is optimal for pregnancy outcome. It remains to be determined whether embryos derived from LH-deficient macaques may undergo asynchronous or delayed development in vivo that could lead to a decreased frequency of implantation.

Are the Midcycle Surges of LH and FSH Redundant Signals? Novel data from the present study demonstrate that a bolus of r-hFSH alone can serve as an ovulatory stimulus to reinitiate nuclear maturation of oocytes capable of

IVF and follicular luteinization at midcycle in macaques receiving a follicular stimulation regimen of r-hFSH. These results are consistent with those from rodent models wherein administration of FSH alone at midcycle can substitute for LH/CG to initiate periovulatory events[9-12]. Since oocytes were recovered at follicle aspiration in the present study, the ability of r-hFSH relative to hCG to induce follicular rupture, i.e. ovulation, was not assessed in the nonhuman primate model. However, ovulation was documented by recovery of oocytes from the oviducts of rodents after a bolus of r-hFSH[9-12] with associated increases in ovarian tissue-type plasminogen activator activity, a potential participant in follicular rupture[34].

Although a midcycle surge of FSH promoted early events in granulosa cell luteinization such as acute production of progesterone and vascular endothelial growth factor as well as expression of nuclear progesterone receptors, it was inadequate to sustain normal luteal function in primates. Whether production of luteal-derived, non-steroidogenic factors is altered in a similar fashion to progesterone after substitution of the midcycle gonadotropin surge with FSH alone is not presently known. Likewise, it is not clear whether the premature decline in progesterone production following r-hFSH administration at midcycle would have physiological relevance for establishing pregnancy in primates.

Although LH receptors reside on both granulosa and theca cells of the mature preovulatory follicle, FSH receptors reside exclusively on granulosa cells[35,36]. Thus, the granulosa cells may play a predominant role during early events of luteinization as well as ovulation in the primate follicle, with a lesser role, if any, of theca cells in promoting these events. Alternatively, a bolus of FSH may stimulate granulosa cell responses that alter thecal function in a paracrine manner during luteinization as demonstrated in the rat[28,29]. Evidence that FSH deprivation via neutralization with FSH antiserum in vivo during midfollicular phase in bonnet monkeys prevented in vitro responsiveness of both granulosa cells to FSH and theca cells to LH supports this mechanism in primates[37].

During spontaneous ovarian cycles in primates, it is not known whether FSH and LH act in concert during the midcycle gonadotropin surge, or are redundant signals to ensure periovulatory events occur.

Our data in gonadotropin-stimulated macaques support the hypothesis that granulosa cells display different functional responses when exposed to low versus high intracellular concentrations of cAMP; the former stimulated primarily by FSH to evoke follicular growth, maturation and estradiol production, and the latter to elicit periovulatory events regardless of the gonadotropin stimulus[38].

Summary

In chronically gonadotropin-deficient macaques, exogenous FSH alone is sufficient to produce growth and maturation of antral follicles which, following an ovulatory stimulus of hCG, yield mature oocytes capable of fertilization and subsequent embryonic development that can ultimately result in live offspring.

While the presence of LH with FSH in a 1:1 ratio during follicular stimulation may impair gametogenic events, exposure to LH may enhance embryo viability and developmental rates, resulting in closer synchrony to the implantation window. Further studies are required to titrate the interval and amount of LH needed during follicular development for optimal post-fertilization events in primates.

A bolus of FSH can substitute for LH/CG as an ovulatory stimulus following follicular stimulation protocols utilizing r-hFSH alone, leading to oocyte maturation, fertilization and early events in follicular luteinization in primates. Thus, the surges of FSH and LH that occur spontaneously at midcycle may be redundant signals to insure that early periovulatory events occur. Whether a midcycle "FSH surge" can evoke ovulation, i.e. rupture of the follicle wall and oocyte release, in primates is not known. The efficacy of an exclusively FSH regimen in IVF-related cycles in producing normal embryonic development and live offspring also awaits investigation. Nonetheless, follicular stimulation/ovulation induction regimens composed solely of FSH offer potential clinical utility for improving fertility in women with polycystic ovarian syndrome, avoiding systemic/local allergic reactions to urinary FSH preparations[39] and reducing infertility in patients with ovarian failure due to LH insensitivity[40].

Acknowledgments

The authors acknowledge and appreciate the numerous contributions of Dr. Jim S. Hutchison as a collaborator and liaison with Ares-Serono throughout these studies. We also thank associates in the Assisted Reproductive Technology Core Laboratory, Dr. David Hess and technicians in the Endocrine Services Core Laboratory, members of the surgical team and animal technicians in the Division of Animal Resources for their expertise.

This work was supported by Ares Advanced Technology, Inc., a member of the Ares-Serono group of companies, and NIH grants HD22400 (to R.L.S.) and RR00163.

References

1. Gore-Langton R.E., Armstrong D.E.: Follicular steroidogenesis and its control. In: Knobil E., Neill J. (eds), *The Physiology of Reproduction.* Raven Press, New York, pp. 571-627, 1994.
2. Porchet H.C., Le Cotonnec J.-Y., Canali S., Zanolo G.: Pharmacokinetics of recombinant human follicle stimulating hormone after intravenous, intramuscular and subcutaneous administration in monkeys, and comparison with intravenous administration of urinary follicle stimulating hormone. Drug Metab. *Disposition*, 21:144-150, 1993.
3. Porchet H.C., Le Cotonnec J.-Y., Neutboom B., Canali S., Zanolo G.: Pharmacokinetics of recombinant human luteinizing hormone after intravenous, intramuscular and subcutaneous administration in monkeys, and comparison with intravenous administration of pituitary luteinizing hormone. *J. Clin. Endocrinol. Metab.*, 80:667-673, 1995.
4. Hoff J.D., Quigley M.E., Yen S.S.C.: Hormonal dynamics at midcycle: a reevaluation. *J. Clin. Endocrinol. Metab.*, 57:792-796, 1983.
5. Weick R.F., Dierschke D.J., Karsch F.J., Butler W.R., Hotchkiss J., Knobil E.: Periovulatory time courses of circulating gonadotropic and ovarian hormones in the rhesus monkey. *Endocrinology*, 93:1140-1147, 1973.
6. Lostroh A.J., Johnson R.E.: Amounts of interstitial cell-stimulating hormone and follicle-stimulating hormone required for follicular development, uterine growth and ovulation in the hypophysectomized rat. *Endocrinology*, 79:991-996, 1966.
7. Harrington F.E., Elton R.L.: Induction of ovulation in adult rats with follicle stimulating hormone. *Proc. Soc. Exp. Biol. Med.*, 132:841-844, 1969.
8. Sogn J.H., Curry Jr T.E., Brannstrom M., Lemaire W.J., Koos R.D., Papkoff H., Janson P.O.: Inhibition of follicle-stimulating hormone-induced ovulation by indomethacin in the perfused rat ovary. *Biol. Reprod.*, 36:536-542, 1987.
9. Galway A.B., Hsueh A.J.W., Keene J.L., Yamoto M., Fauser B.C.J.M., Boime I.: In vitro and in vivo bioactivity of recombinant human follicle-stimulating hormone and partially deglycosylated variants secreted by transfected eukaryotic cell lines. *Endocrinology*, 127:93-100, 1990.
10. Tapanainen J.S., LaPolt P.S., Perlas E., Hsueh A.J.W.: Induction of ovarian follicle luteinization by recombinant follicle-stimulating hormone. *Endocrinology*, 133:2875-2880, 1993.
11. Wang X.-N., Greenwald G.S.: Human chorionic gonadotropin or human recombinant follicle stimulating hormone (FSH)-induced ovulation and subsequent fertilization and early embryo development in hypophysect-

omized FSH-primed mice. *Endocrinology*, 132:2009-2016, 1993.
12. Montgomery-Rice V., Loutradis D., Tulchinsky D., Kiessling A.: FSH-induced ovulation in intact and hypophysectomized mice. *J. Reprod. Fertil.*, 84:1-6, 1988.
13. Zelinski-Wooten M.B., Hutchison J.S., Hess D.L., Wolf D.P., Stouffer R.L.: Follicle stimulating hormone alone supports follicle growth and oocyte development in gonadotrophin-releasing hormone antagonist-treated monkeys. *Hum. Reprod.*, 10:1658-1666, 1995.
14. Gougeon A.: Dynamics of follicular growth in the human: a model from preliminary results. *Hum. Reprod.*, 1:81-87, 1986.
15. Wolf D.P., Thomson J.A., Zelinski-Wooten M.B., Stouffer R.L.: In vitro fertilization-embryo transfer in nonhuman primates: the technique and its applications. *Mol. Reprod. Dev.*, 27:261-280, 1990.
16. Weston A.M., Zelinski-Wooten M.B., Hutchison J.S., Stouffer R.L., Wolf D.P.: Developmental potential of embryos produced by in-vitro fertilization from gonadotrophin-releasing hormone antagonist-treated macaques stimulated with recombinant human follicle stimulating hormone alone or in combination with luteinizing hormone. *Hum. Reprod.*, 11:608-613, 1996.
17. Zelinski-Wooten M.B., Hutchison J.S., Trinchard-Lugan I., Hess D.L., Wolf D.P., Stouffer R.L.: Initiation of periovulatory events in gonadotrophin-stimulated macaques with varying doses of recombinant human chorionic gonadotropin. *Hum. Reprod.*, 12:1877-1885, 1997.
18. Zelinski-Wooten M.B., Hutchison J.S., Hess D.L., Wolf D.P., Stouffer R.L.: A bolus of recombinant human follicle stimulating hormone at midcycle induces periovulatory events following multiple follicular development in macaques. *Hum. Reprod.*, 13:554-560, 1998.
19. Aladin Chandrasekher Y., Brenner R.M., Molskness T.A., Yu Q., Stouffer R.L.: Titrating luteinizing hormone surge requirements for ovulatory changes in primate follicles. II. Progesterone receptor expression in luteinizing granulosa cells. *J. Clin. Endocrinol. Metab.*, 73:584-589, 1991.
20. Christenson L.K., Stouffer R.L.: Follicle-stimulating hormone and luteinizing hormone/chorionic gonadotropin stimulation of vascular endothelial growth factor production by macaque granulosa cells from pre- and periovulatory follicles. *J. Clin. Endocrinol. Metab.*, 82:2135-2142, 1997.
21. Kenigsberg D., Littman B.A., Williams R.F., Hodgen G.D.: Medical hypophysectomy: II. Variability of ovarian response to gonadotropin therapy. *Fertil. Steril.*, 42:116-126, 1984.
22. Couzinet B., Lestrat N., Brailly S., Forest M., Schaison G.: Stimulation of ovarian follicular maturation with pure follicle-stimulating hormone in women with gonadotropin deficiency. *J. Clin. Endocrinol. Metab.*, 66:552-

556, 1988.
23. Shoham Z., Balen A., Patel A., Jacobs H.S.: Results of ovulation induction using human menopausal gonadotropin or purified follicle-stimulating hormone in hypogonadotrophic hypogonadism patients. *Fertil. Steril.*, 56: 1048-1053, 1991.
24. Schoot D.C., Bennink H.J.T.C., Mannaerts B.M.J.L., Lamberts S.W.J., Bouchard P., Fauser B.C.J.M.: Human recombinant follicle-stimulating hormone induces growth of preovulatory follicles without concomitant increase in androgen and estrogen biosynthesis in a woman with isolated gonadotropin deficiency. *J. Clin. Endocrinol. Metab.*, 74:1471-1473, 1992.
25. Shoham Z., Mannaerts B., Insler V., Coelingh-Bennink H.: Induction of follicular growth using recombinant human follicle-stimulating hormone in two volunteer women with hypogonadotrophic hypogonadism. *Fertil. Steril.*, 59:738-742, 1993.
26. Karnitis V.J., Townson D.H., Friedman C.I., Danforth D.R.: Recombinant human follicle-stimulating hormone stimulates multiple follicular growth, but minimal estrogen production in gonadotropin-releasing hormone antagonist-treated monkeys: examining the role of luteinizing hormone (LH) in follicular development and steroidogenesis. *J. Clin. Endocrinol. Metab.*, 79:91-97, 1994.
27. Chappel S.C., Howles C.: Reevaluation of the roles of luteinizing hormone and follicle-stimulating hormone in the ovulatory process. *Hum. Reprod.*, 6:1206-1212, 1991.
28. Hillier S.G., Smyth C.D., Whitelaw P.F., Miro F., Howles C.: Gonadotrophin control of follicular function. *Horm. Res*, 43:216-223, 1995.
29. Smyth C.D., Miro F., Howles C.M., Hillier S.G.: Effect of luteinizing hormone on follicle stimulating hormone-activated paracrine signalling in rat ovary. *Hum. Reprod.*, 10:33-39, 1995.
30. Baird D.T., Campbell B.K.: Supplementation with recombinant LH to reduce multiple folliculogenesis and ovarian hyperstimulation. In: Filicori M., Flamigni C. (ed.), *Ovulation Induction Update '98*. Parthenon Publishing Group, New York, pp. 159-168, 1998.
31. Balasch J., Miro F., Burzaco I., Casamitjana R., Civico S., Ballesca J.L., Puerto B., Vanrell J.A.: The role of luteinizing hormone in human follicle development and oocyte fertility: evidence from in-vitro fertilization in a woman with long-standing hypogonadotrophic hypogonadism and using recombinant human follicle stimulating hormone. *Hum. Reprod.*, 10:1678-1683, 1995.
32. Zelinski-Wooten M.B., Stouffer R.L.: Steroids receptors and action in the primate follicle. *Trends Endocrinol. Metab.*, 7:177-183, 1996.

33. Iskovitz-Eldor J., Kol S., Mannaerts, Coelingh Bennink H.: First established pregnancy after controlled ovarian hyperstimulation with recombinant follicle stimulating hormone and the gonadotrophin-releasing hormone antagonist ganirelix (Org 37462). *Hum. Reprod.*, 13:294-295, 1998.
34. Galway A.B., LaPolt P.S., Tsafriri A., Dargan C.M., Boime I., Hsueh A.J.W.: Recombinant follicle-stimulating hormone induces ovulation and tissue plasminogen activator expression in hypophysetomized rats. *Endocrinology*, 127:3023-3028, 1990.
35. Kobayashi M., Nakano R., Ooshima A.: Immunocytochemical localization of pituitary gonadotrophins and gonadal steroids confirms the 'two-cell, two-gonadotropin' hypothesis of steroidogenesis in the human ovary. *J. Endocrinol.*, 126:483-488, 1990.
36. Yamamoto M., Shima K., Nakano R.: Gonadotropin receptors in human ovarian follicles and corpora lutea throughout the menstrual cycle. *Horm. Res*, 37 (Suppl. 1):5-11, 1992.
37. Selvaraj N., Moudgal N.R.: In vivo and in vitro studies on the differential role of luteinizing hormone and follicle-stimulating hormone in regulating follicular function in the bonnet monkey *(Macaca radiata)* using specific gonadotropin antibodies. *Biol. Reprod.*, 51:246-253.
38. Yong E.L., Baird D.T., Hillier S.G.: Mediation of gonadotrophin-stimulated growth and differentiation of human granulosa cells by adenosine-3',5'-monophosphate: one molecule, two messages. *Clin. Endocrinol.*, 37:51-58, 1992.
39. Phipps W.R., Holden D., Sheehan R.K.: Use of recombinant human follicle-stimulating hormone for in vitro fertilization-embryo transfer after severe systemic immunoglobulin E-mediated reaction to urofollitropin. *Fertil. Steril.*, 66:148-150, 1996.
40. Latronico A.C., Anasti J.A., Arnhold I.J.P., Rapaport R., Mendonca B.B., Bloise W., Castro M., Tsigos C., Chrousos G.P.: Testicular and ovarian resistance to luteinizing hormone caused by inactivating mutations of the luteinizing hormone-receptor gene. *N. Engl. J. Med.*, 334:507-512, 1996.

The Role of Luteinizing Hormone
in Folliculogenesis
and Ovulation Induction, pp. 37-51
Editor M. Filicori

Endocrine and Paracrine Control of Oocyte Function

D.R. Danforth, L.K. Arbogast and B. Alak

*Department of Obstetrics and Gynecology,
The Ohio State University, Columbus, Ohio (United States of America)*

Abstract. *The regulation and control of oocyte function are complex processes involving both local (paracrine) and extraovarian (endocrine) factors. Moreover the paracrine regulation of oocyte development is likely under endocrine control. The principal endocrine hormones modulating oocyte development are the gonadotropins LH and FSH. The effects of these gonadotropins on oocyte development may be mediated through a variety of mechanisms, including ovarian production of growth factors, cytokines, inhibins, activins, and steroids. Specific receptors for steroids, growth factors, and cytokines have been demonstrated on oocytes of several species. Gonadotropin modulation of follicular concentrations of these paracrine factors may ultimately be responsible for the precise regulation of oocyte maturation. As GnRH antagonists and recombinant gonadotropins become available, the clinical utility of more precise control of the endocrine, paracrine, and autocrine regulation of follicle growth and oocyte development can be more thoroughly investigated.*

Key words. Gonadotropins, oocytes, paracrine factors, growth factors.

Introduction

The regulation and control of oocyte function is a complex process involving both local (paracrine) and extraovarian (endocrine) factors. Moreover, the paracrine regulation of oocyte development is surely under endocrine control. The principal endocrine hormones modulating oocyte development are likely the gonadotropins luteinizing hormone (LH) and follicle-stimulating hormone (FSH).

It is clear from numerous clinical and basic studies that until midcycle, FSH is the primary gonadotropin responsible for follicle growth and oocyte development in humans and nonhuman primates. Indeed, it is becoming increasingly clear that LH may in fact be detrimental to oocyte development, at least when present in elevated amounts.

There are limited data in the literature suggesting that addition of gonadotropins *in vitro* may also modulate oocyte development. Prins et al.[1] reported that addition of human menopausal gonadotropin (hMG) *in vitro* enhanced maturation and fertilization rates of immature oocytes recovered for in vitro fertilization (IVF). Zhang et al.[2] reported that addition of hMG to human oocytes obtained from small follicles also increased fertilization rates compared with non-hMG-treated oocytes, but not to the levels observed with larger, more mature follicles. In Rhesus monkeys, gonadotropins influence maturation of immature oocytes in a cycle phase dependent manner[3]. Addition of FSH and LH enhance maturation of oocytes recovered during the late follicular and luteal phases, but inhibits completion of meiosis in oocytes recovered during the early follicular phase. In contrast, Durinzi et al.[4] were unable to demonstrate any effect of in vitro addition of FSH on maturation of immature human oocytes, although steroid production was enhanced. Similarly, more detailed experiments on mouse oocytes also suggest a lack of effect or perhaps even a deleterious effect of in vitro addition of FSH to murine oocyte-granulosa cell complexes[5,6]. Thus, there is contradictory evidence for the role of gonadotropins in vitro, although it seems likely that FSH is not required for in vitro maturation of oocytes.

Gonadotropins can affect oocyte development either via direct action on the oocyte or indirectly via the granulosa or theca cells. Since there are no reports to date that demonstrate gonadotropin receptors on oocytes, the reported actions of gonadotropins on oocytes are more likely indirect, via paracrine mediators from granulosa or theca cells or possibly other cells within the ovary. These mediators of gonadotropin action on oocytes include growth factors, steroids, cytokines, the inhibins and activins, and oocyte maturation inhibitor (OMI).

Paracrine Factors and Oocyte Development

Growth Factors. Ovary-produced or peripherally derived growth factors, including epidermal growth factor (EGF), vascular endothelial growth factor (VEGF), insulin-like growth factors I and II (IGF-I, IGF-II), and their binding proteins are becoming recognized as important modulators of many aspects of ovarian function, including growth and selection of the dominant follicle, oocyte development, and corpus luteum function. The demonstration of transcripts for IGF-I and IGF-II receptor[7] and EGF receptor protein[8] in oocytes from human ovaries suggests that the growth factors may be directly involved in oocyte development and maturation. Gomez et al.[9] examined the effects of *in vitro* addition of growth factors on the maturation of oocytes retrieved from unstimulated ovaries in patients who did not receive gonadotropins. Addition of EGF *in vitro* enhanced the rate of germinal vesicle breakdown and oocyte maturation. The effects of IGF were comparable to those observed with EGF. However, these studies were performed with cumulus-oocyte complexes, and it is unknown whether these effects were via direct action on the oocyte or mediated by the granulosa cells. Similar results have been reported for these growth factors in a variety of other species[10-12]. Because ovarian growth factor production is under gonadotropin regulation, gonadotropin stimulation of growth factor and of growth factor binding protein production by granulosa cells may be an important mechanism whereby gonadotropins modulate oocyte function. Moreover, there is a tight communication between cumulus cells and the oocyte via gap junctional complexes, and both gonadotropins and growth factors may influence oocyte development by modulating the direct communication and transfer of mediators from granulosa cells to oocytes.

Ovarian Steroids. Ovarian steroids are another class of potential paracrine mediators of gonadotropin action on oocyte development. The role of steroids on oocyte function has been investigated for many years. Clearly, alteration of the steroidogenic milieu that surrounds the oocyte can have dramatic effects on oocyte function. Classic studies from McNatty et al.[13] indicate that the ratio of intrafollicular androgen to estrogen (A-E) is highly correlated with oocyte status. Follicles with healthy oocytes that have undergone germinal vesicle (GV) breakdown have the lowest A-E ratio. Follicles that contain intact GVs but degenerating oocytes have an intermediate A-E ratio, and follicles that are overtly necrotic have the highest A-E ratio. These data suggest that the intrafollicular androgen and estrogen environment is highly correlated with, and may be a good predictor of oocyte function.

More recently, Zelinski-Wooten et al. have directly manipulated androgen and/or estradiol levels using an aromatase inhibitor[14] or a 3ß-hydroxy-steroid dehydrogenase (3ß-HSD) inhibitor[15]. Both compounds significantly inhibit peripheral estradiol levels and, by inference, intrafollicular estradiol concentrations in gonadotropin-stimulated monkeys. Acute elevation of androgen: estrogen ratios by inhibition of aromatase results in an increase in the number of immature oocytes recovered, a decrease in the number of oocytes reaching metaphase II, and a decrease in the fertilization rate of these oocytes (Table 1)[14]. In contrast, suppression of estradiol without a concomitant increase in

TABLE 1 - *Characteristics of oocytes collected from gonadotropin-stimulated rhesus monkeys after follicular maturation in the presence or absence of an aromatase inhibitor (ATD).*

Oocyte maturation and performance	*Control*	*ATD*
No. of ova/animal (mean ± SEM)	34±7	30±7
Prophase I (%)	11	31*
MI (%)	58	60
MII (%)	26	4*
Atretic (%)	6	5
No. inseminated	78	65
No. fertilized	32	6*
Fertilization rate (%)	25	9*
Cleavage rate (%)	94	100

Adapted with permission from Zelinski-Wooten et al.[14]
MI, Metaphase I; MII, metaphase II.
*Different ($p < 0.05$) from controls within row.

androgen concentrations (as observed with inhibition of 3ß-HSD) had no effect on oocyte maturation; however, fertilization rates were reduced in 3 of 4 monkeys[15]. Interestingly, in both studies, the decrease in ovarian estradiol production had no effect on follicle growth. These data suggest that decreased follicular estradiol production and increased androgen-estrogen ratios may impair oocyte development and fertilization ability in these nonhuman primates.

It is likely that estradiol is a direct modulator of oocyte function. Using rtPCR, Wu et al.[16] demonstrated estrogen receptor message in human oocytes (Figure 1). In contrast, relatively little estrogen receptor is expressed in the cumulus cells surrounding the oocytes, and other investigators have demonstrated a relative lack of estrogen receptors in granulosa and theca cells of primate ovaries[17]. These data are consistent with the observation that estradiol directly modulates oocyte function but has relatively little effect on follicle growth in humans and in nonhuman primates. However, the recent identification of a second form of the estrogen receptor (ERß) may provide new insights into the role of estradiol on oocyte function and follicle development. Byers et al.[18] has demonstrated that the rat ovary expresses both ERα and ERß genes, but ERß is the predominant form of the estrogen receptor in the rat ovary. Similarly, Duffy et al.[19] recently reported differential expression of ERß but not ERα mRNA in ovulatory follicles of the monkey ovary. The presence of ERß in oocytes has yet to be reported.

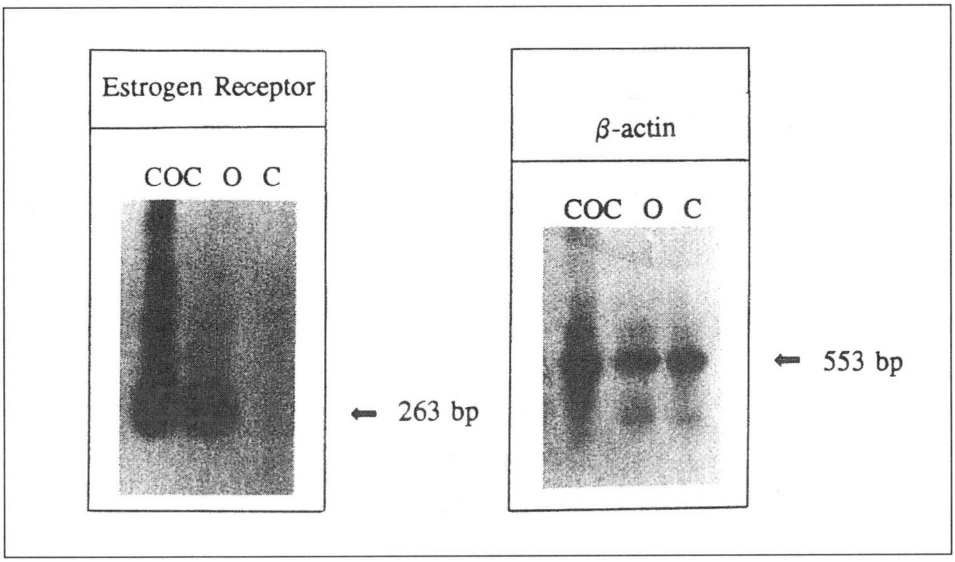

FIGURE 1 - *Confirmation of amplified cDNA products for estrogen receptors (ER). Total RNA extracted from five human cumulus-oocyte complexes (COC), oocytes (O), and cumulus masses (C) was used in reverse transcriptase polymerase chain reaction for amplification of ER (left) and β-actin (right) cDNAs. After agarose gel electrophoresis, the amplified products were transferred to nylon membrane for Southern blot hybridization with 32P-labeled ER or β-actin cDNA probes* (adapted with permission from Wu et al.[16]).

In addition to the possible effects of ERß-mediated estrogen action on oocytes, the non-genomic effects of estrogen and other steroids on reproductive tissues is becoming better understood (for review see 20). Estradiol can induce a rapid (within seconds) increase in Ca++ influx in human oocytes[21], and this effect is antagonized by androgens[22]. Tesarik et al.[21,22] propose that estradiol exerts a beneficial effect on cytoplasmic maturation via a non-genomic calcium-mediated mechanism, and that the estrogen/androgen environment of the developing follicle affects oocyte quality via non-genomic pathways.

Although marked reduction in ovarian estradiol production and an increased follicular androgen to estrogen ratio may be detrimental to oocyte function, supraphysiologic elevation of estradiol levels may also adversely affect oocyte development, fertilization, and/or ultimate pregnancy outcome. Certainly, supraphysiologic levels of estradiol as obtained in ovulation induction or IVF protocols may advance the age of the endometrium and narrow the window of opportunity for implantation. Moreover, through a variety of mechanisms, elevated LH levels have also been associated with decreased oocyte function and decreased pregnancy outcome.

Cytokines. In recent years, there has been increased interest in the role of cytokines in reproductive medicine. A variety of cytokines have been reported to modulate hypothalamic and pituitary function, and they may have direct effects on the ovarian follicle and modulate corpus luteum function. Although few studies that investigate cytokine regulation of oocyte development have been performed, the type 1 receptor for interleukin-1 was recently detected in high abundance in murine oocytes[23] and secretion of various cytokines by oocytes or cumulus-oocyte complexes has been reported[24]. Moreover, the dramatic effects of cytokines on granulosa and theca cell function and their

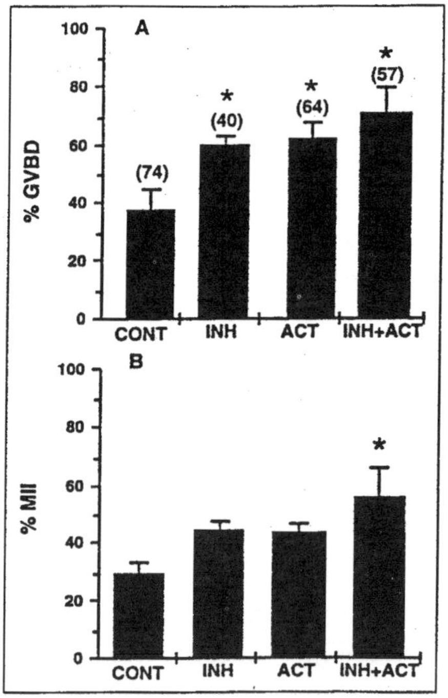

FIGURE 2 - *Effect of inhibin (INH), activin (ACT) or INH + ACT on Rhesus monkey oocyte maturation in vitro expressed as a percentage of the total number of oocytes that A) underwent GVBD, or B) reached MII after 48h of culture.* (From Alak, et al.[26]).

regulation by gonadotropins suggest that this class of compounds may play an important role in modulating oocyte function as well.

Inhibins/Activins. Another family of hormones that may modulate oocyte development is the inhibins and activins. In addition to their postulated roles in regulating circulating FSH, it appears that these hormones have paracrine actions in the ovary that regulate follicular growth and oocyte function. The dramatic effects of activin on follicle development in vitro underscores the potential important paracrine role of this "hormone" in the ovary[25]. Recent data suggest that the inhibins and activins may also participate in oocyte maturation. Activin stimulates meiotic maturation of bovine oocytes[26] *in vitro.* Similarly, addition of inhibin and/or activin *in vitro* results in stimulation of germinal vesicle breakdown and maturation to metaphase II of cumulus-oocyte complexes obtained from monkeys (Figure 2)[27]. Addition of follistatin blocks the stimulating effect of activin. Likewise, activin stimulated meiotic maturation of human[28] oocytes (Figure 3), and modulates granulosa cell steroidogenesis.

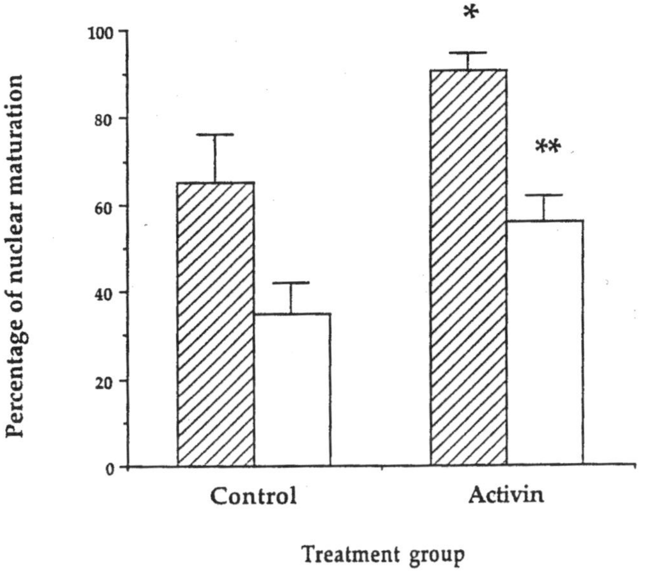

FIGURE 3 - *Effect of activin-A on human oocyte maturation in vitro. Oocyte maturation is expressed as the percentage of the total number of oocytes that underwent germinal vessicle breakdown (striped bar) or reached MII (open bar) after 48h of culture. Statistically different from control values, *P<0.005, **P<0.001.* (From Alak et al., in press[28]).

Oocyte maturation inhibitor. It has been recognized for many years that oocytes spontaneously resume meiosis *in vitro* once removed from the follicular environment. It has therefore been suggested that an endogenous OMI that maintains the oocyte in meiotic arrest is present *in vivo.*

Although a number of candidates have been proposed for this molecule, the difficulty in establishing and reproducing *in vitro* oocyte maturation assays has hampered progress toward conclusive identification of this substance. One of the more promising candidates is cyclic adenosine monophosphate (cAMP). Addition of cAMP *in vitro* inhibits resumption of oocyte maturation, and depletion of cAMP levels within oocytes allows meiosis to resume[29]. Cyclic AMP levels within oocytes *in vivo* may be regulated by gonadotropin modulation of cumulus cell-oocyte gap junctions, altering the movement of cAMP from granulosa cells to oocytes and vice versa.

Gonadotropins as Endocrine Regulators of Oocyte Development and Ovulation

The Role of Gonadotropins in Follicle Growth and Oocyte Development. To investigate the relative roles of FSH, LH, and estradiol on follicle growth[30] and oocyte function[31], we and others have utilized gonadotropin-releasing hormone (GnRH) antagonists (to suppress endogenous pituitary function) combined with recombinant (pure) gonadotropins for ovulation induction in nonhuman primates. In the absence of endogenous gonadotropin support, administration of recombinant FSH resulted in a tenfold reduction in circulating estradiol levels as compared with hMG-treated animals, which is likely due to a lack of LH-stimulated androgen precursor production by the theca cells (Figure 4). However, follicle growth was similar in the hMG- and recombinant FSH-treated monkeys, which indicates that robust follicular growth can be obtained without supraphysiologic estradiol production.

Using a similar GnRH antagonist-treated primate model, Zelinski-Wooten et al.[31] demonstrated that monkeys treated with recombinant FSH had significantly fewer immature oocytes, more mature oocytes, and an increased fertilization rate as compared with monkeys treated with FSH plus LH (Table 2). However, the developmental potential of the embryos (cryosurvival and development in vitro) is slightly greater for the FSH+LH treated monkeys[32]. Thus, it may be beneficial to stimulate multiple follicular growth while maintaining relatively physiologic estradiol concentrations, not only for oocyte quality but also for a more appropriate endometrial priming. Moreover, the data are consistent with the hypothesis that intraovarian steroid concentrations play an important role in modulating oocyte development. These preclinical studies

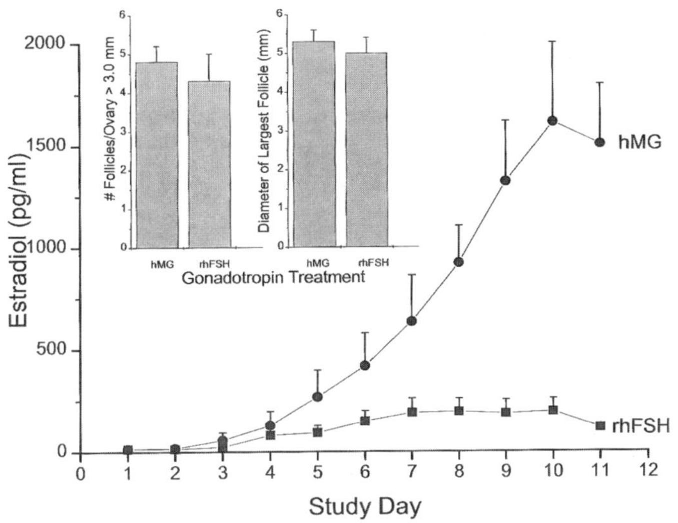

FIGURE 4 - *Serum estradiol levels and follicle growth (inset) in cynomolgus monkeys treated with GnRH antagonist plus gonadotropins for ovulation induction. Monkeys were treated with hMG or rhFSH as indicated on the figure.* (From Karnitis et al.[30]).

have been extended by a variety of clinical data evaluating recombinant (pure) FSH for ovulation induction in ART cycles which will be reviewed elsewhere in these proceedings.

The Role of Gonadotropins in Final Oocyte Maturation. In the natural cycle, surges of both LH and FSH occur at midcycle, but LH is certainly the primary gonadotropin responsible for final oocyte maturation and ovulation.

TABLE 2 - *Gonadotropin effects on oocyte development.*

Oocyte maturation and performance	*rhFSH*	*rhFSH + rhLH (1:1)*
Prophase I (%)	2	15
MII (%)	39	16
Fertilization rate (%)	90	43

Adapted with permission from Zelinski-Wooten et al.[31]

Recombinant DNA-derived LH[33,34], purified human urinary LH[35], and hCG[36] induce ovulation and/or oocyte maturation in gonadotropin-stimulated monkeys. In addition, hCG is routinely used as the ovulatory stimulus in ovulation induction and IVF protocols. However, recent evidence suggests that FSH may also be able to substitute for LH (or hCG) as the ovulatory stimulus. Recombinant FSH stimulates follicle growth and induces ovulation in hypophysectomized rats[37], and oocytes from FSH-ovulated animals will fertilize and undergo apparently normal fetal development[38]. Similarly, rhFSH is equivalent to rhCG for oocyte maturation and fertilization in gonadotropin stimulated monkeys[39]. The clinical utility of FSH-induced ovulation, for example to potentially reduce the risk of ovarian hyperstimulation syndrome, remains to be investigated.

An important issue when considering ovulation-induction agents is the strength vs the duration of the ovulatory stimulus. In primates, the typical midcycle gonadotropin surge lasts 48 to 50 hours, considerably longer than the 10- to 16-hour surge observed in domestic animals. This prolonged elevation of LH and prolonged exposure of the granulosa cells and oocyte to the ovulatory stimulus are important for completion of oocyte maturation and luteinization of granulosa cells. Monkeys treated with a single GnRH injection to induce LH surge (after gonadotropin stimulation of follicle growth) manifest a surge comparable in height to the typical midcycle LH surge but one that lasts for only 4 to 6 hours[40]. Oocytes retrieved from these animals are mostly immature (GV intact). Moreover, adequate luteinization of granulosa cells also fails to occur in these animals. These and other data[34,36] indicate that the duration of the ovulatory stimulus is at least as important as the height of the surge and may have implications in clinical practice as GnRH, GnRH analogues, and recombinant gonadotropins are considered for triggering ovulation or final oocyte maturation.

LH Hypersecretion and the Oocyte. In the past decade, significant attention has been focused on the adverse effects of elevated LH on oocyte function[41,42]. The results of a majority of studies are consistent with the hypothesis that hypersecretion of LH during follicular growth is associated with a poor outcome, including poor fertilization and pregnancy rates and increased rates of spontaneous abortion. However, other data have failed to confirm the correlation between elevated LH and pregnancy outcome[43,44]. The adverse effects of elevated LH could be mediated by excess production by the ovary of steroids, growth factors, inhibins and activins, and cytokines. Alternatively, adverse effects on the endometrium and premature resumption of meiosis may contribute to the negative sequelae associated with hypersecretion of LH.

Recent data suggest that the effects of hypersecretion of LH are not mediated via endometrial or uterine effects but are primarily of ovarian origin[45].

The evidence supporting the correlation between premature resumption of meiosis and elevated LH is most persuasive. Elevated LH levels may lead to premature expansion of the cumulus cells, which results in loss of intimate contact between the oocytes and the cumulus cells. Consequently, the transfer of OMI (or other factors) from granulosa cells to oocytes is decreased, allowing the oocytes to resume meiosis prematurely. This process results in the ovulation or retrieval of postmature oocytes that demonstrate subnormal fertilization and developmental ability. Thus, the retrieval or the ovulation of postmature oocytes may be the end product of hypersecretion of LH during follicle growth.

Conclusions

The effects of gonadotropins on oocyte development are most likely mediated through a variety of mechanisms, including granulosa cell production of growth factors, cytokines, inhibins and activins, and steroids. In pathophysiologic situations, such as hypersecretion of LH, premature resumption of meiosis and excess androgen production may have a negative impact on oocyte function. At the other end of the spectrum, the absence or reduction of LH (in gonadotropin-deficient or GnRH antagonist-treated patients) may improve oocyte quality by decreasing intrafollicular androgen and estrogen levels and allowing synchronous final maturation of oocytes. Indeed, as GnRH antagonists and recombinant gonadotropins become widely utilized, the clinical usefulness of more precise control of endocrine, paracrine, and autocrine regulation of follicle growth and oocyte development can be investigated more thoroughly.

References

1. Prins G.S., Wagner C., Weidel L., Gianfortoni J., Marut E.L., Scommegna A.: Gonadotropins augment maturation and fertilization of human immature oocytes cultured in vitro. *Fertil. Steril.*, 47:1035-1037, 1987.
2. Zhang X., Zerafa A., Wong J., Armstrong D.T., Khamsi F.: Human menopausal gonadotropin during in vitro maturation of human oocytes retrieved from small follicles enhances in vitro fertilization and cleavage rates. *Fertil. Steril.*, 59:850-853. 1993.
3. Alak B.M., Wolf D.P.: Rhesus monkey oocyte maturation and fertilization *in vitro*: roles of menstrual cycle phase and of exogenous gonadotropins.

Biol. Reprod., 51:879-887, 1994.
4. Durinzi K.L., Wentz A.C., Saniaga E.M., Johnson D.E., Lazendorf S.E.: Follicle stimulating hormone effects on unstimulated human oocytes: in vitro maturation and hormone production. *J. Assisted Reprod. Genetics.*, 14:199-204, 1997.
5. Eppig J.J., O'Brien M.J.: Development in vitro of mouse oocytes from primordial follicles. *Biol. Reprod.*, 54:197-207, 1996.
6. Eppig J.J., O'Brien M.J., Pendola F.L.: Oocyte development in vitro [Abstract M-15]. In: *Proceedings of the 31st Meeting of the Society for the Study of Reproduction*, College Station, Texas, August 8-11, 1998.
7. Zhou J., Bondy C.: Anatomy of the human ovarian insulin-like growth factor system. *Biol. Reprod.*, 48:467-482, 1993.
8. Maruo T., Ladines-Llave C.A., Samoto T., et al.: Expression of epidermal growth factor and its receptor in the human ovary during follicular growth and regression. *Endocrinology*, 132:924-931, 1993.
9. Gomez E., Tarin J.J., Pellicer A.: Oocyte maturation in humans: the role of gonadotropins and growth factors. *Fertil. Steril.*, 60:40-46, 1993.
10. Das K., Stout L.E., Hensleigh H.C., Tagatz G.E., Phipps W.R., Leung B.S.: Direct positive effect of epidermal growth factor on the cytoplasmic maturation of mouse and human oocytes. *Fertil. Steril.*, 55:1000-1004, 1991.
11. Feng P., Catt K.J., Knecht M.: Transforming growth factor-ß stimulates meiotic maturation of the rat oocyte. *Endocrinology*, 122:181-186, 1988.
12. Coskun S., Lin Y.C.: Site of action of epidermal growth factor (EGF) on in vitro porcine oocyte maturation. *Endocr. J.*, 1:87-91, 1993.
13. McNatty K.P., Moore Smith D., Makris A., Osathanondh R., Ryan K.J.: The microenvironment of the human antral follicle: interrelationships among the steroid levels in antral fluid, and population of granulosa cells, and the status of the oocyte in vivo and in vitro. *J. Clin. Endocrinol. Metab.*, 49:851-860, 1979.
14. Zelinski-Wooten M.B., Hess D.L., Baughman W.L., Molskness T.A., Wolf D.P., Stouffer R.L.: Administration of an aromatase inhibitor during the late follicular phase of gonadotropin-treated cycles in rhesus monkeys: effects on follicle development, oocyte maturation, and subsequent luteal function. *J. Clin. Endocrinol. Metab.*, 76:988-995, 1993.
15. Zelinski-Wooten M.B., Hess D.L., Wolf D.P., Stouffer R.L.: Steroid reduction during ovarian stimulation impairs oocyte fertilization, but not folliculogenesis, in rhesus monkeys. *Fertil. Steril.*, 61:1147-1155, 1994.
16. Wu T.C.J., Wang L., Wan Y.J.Y.: Detection of estrogen receptor messenger ribonucleic acid in human oocytes and cumulus-oocyte complexes using reverse transcriptase-polymerase chain reaction. *Fertil. Steril.*, 59:54-59,

1993.
17. Hild-Petito S., Stouffer R.L., Brenner R.M.: Immunocytochemical localization of estradiol and progesterone receptors in the monkey ovary throughout the menstrual cycle. *Endocrinology,* 123:2896-2905, 1988.
18. Byers M., Kuiper G.G.J.M., Gustafsson J.A., Park-Sarge O.K.: Estrogen receptor-ß mRNA expression in rat ovary: down-reguation by gonadotropins. *Mol. Endocrinol.,* 11:172-182, 1997.
19. Duffy D.M., Stouffer L., Chaffin C.L.: Noncoordinated expression of estrogen α and ß in the ovulatory follicle and the corpus luteum of the rhesus monkey [Abstract 118]. In: *Proceedings of the 31st Meeting of the Society for the Study of Reproduction,* College Station, Texas, August 8-11, 1998.
20. Revelli A., Massobrio M., Tesarik J.: Nongenomic actions of steroid hormones in reproductive tissues. *Endocr. Rev.,* 19:3-17, 1998.
21. Tesarik J., Mendoza C.: Nongenomic effects of 17(-estradiol on maturing human oocytes: relationship to oocyte developmental potential. *J. Clin. Endocrinol. Metab.,* 80:1438-1443, 1995.
22. Tesarik J., Mendoza C.: Direct non-genomic effects of folicular steroids on maturing human oocytes: oestrogen vs. androgen antagonism. *Hum. Reprod. Update,* 3:95-100, 1997.
23. Simon C., Frances A., Piquette G., Polan M.L.: Immunohistochemical localization of the interleukin-1 system in the mouse ovary during follicular growth, ovulation, and luteinization. *Biol. Reprod.,* 50:449-457, 1994.
24. Zolti M., Ben-Rafael Z., Meiron R., Shemesh M., Bider D., Mashiach S., Apte R.: Cytokine involvement in oocytes and early embryos. *Fertil. Steril.,* 56:265-272, 1991.
25. Li R., Phillips D.M., Mather J.P.: Activin promotes ovarian follicle development in vitro. *Endocrinology,* 136:849-956, 1995.
26. Stock A.E., Woodruff T.K., Smith L.C.: Effects of inhibin A and activin A during in vitro maturation of bovine oocytes in hormone- and serum-free medium. *Biol. Reprod.,* 56:1559-1564, 1997.
27. Alak B.M., Smith G.D., Woodruff T.K., Stouffer R.L., Wolf D.P.: Enhancement of primate oocyte maturation and fertilization in vitro by inhibin A and activin A. *Fertil. Steril.,* 66:646-653, 1996.
28. Alak B.M., Coskun S., Friedman C.I., Kennard E.A., Kim M.H., Seifer D.B.: Activin-A stimulates maturation of human oocytes and modulates granulosa cell steroidogenensis in vitro. *Fertil. Steril.,* In press.
29. Schultz R.M., Montgomery R.R., Belanoff J.R.: Regulation of mouse oocyte meiotic maturation: implication of a decrease in oocyte cAMP and protein dephosphorylation in commitment to resume meiosis. *Dev. Biol.,* 97:264-273, 1983.

30. Karnitis V.J., Townson D.L., Friedman C.I., Danforth D.R.: Recombinant human follicle stimulating hormone stimulates multiple follicular growth but minimal estrogen production in gonadotropin releasing hormone antagonist treated monkeys: examining the role of luteinizing hormone in follicular development and steroidogenesis. *J. Clin. Endocrinol. Metab.*, 79:91-97, 1994.
31. Zelinski-Wooten M.B., Hutchison J.S., Hess D.L., Wolf D.P., Stouffer R.L.: Follicle stimulating hormone alone supports follicle growth and oocyte development in gonadotrophin-releasing hormone antagonist-treated monkeys. *Hum. Reprod.*, 10:1658-1666, 1995.
32. Weston A.M., Zelinski-Wooten M.B., Hutchison J.S., Stouffer R.L., Wolf D.P.: Developmental potential of embryos produced by in-vitro fertilization from gonadotrophin-releasing hormone antagonist-treated macaques stimulated with recombinant human follicle stimulating hormone alone or in combination with luteinizing hormone. *Hum. Reprod.*, 11:608-613, 1996.
33. Simon J.A., Danforth D.R., Hutchison J.S., Hodgen G.D.: Characterization of recombinant DNA derived human luteinizing hormone in vitro and in vivo: efficacy in ovulation induction and corpus luteum support. *J.A.M.A.*, 259:3290-3295, 1988.
34. Chandrasekher Y.A., Hutchison J.S., Zelinski-Wooten M.B., Hess D.L., Wolf D.P., Stouffer R.L.: Initiation of periovulatory events in primate follicles using recombinant and native luteinizing hormone to mimic the midcycle gonadotropin surge. *J. Clin. Endocrinol. Metab.*, 79(1):298-306, 1994.
35. Zelinski-Wooten M.B., Hutchison J.S., Chandrasekher Y.A., Wolf D.P., Stouffer R.L.: Administration of human luteinizing hormone (hLH) to macaques after follicular development: further titration of LH surge requirements for ovulatory changes in primate follicles. *J. Clin. Endocrinol. Metab.*, 75:502-507, 1992.
36. Zelinski-Wooten M.B., Hutchison J.S., Trinchard-Lugan I., Hess D.L., Wolf D.P., Stouffer R.L.: Initiation of periovulatory events in gonadotrophin-stimulated macaques with varying doses of recombinant human chorionic gonadotrophin. *Hum. Reprod.*, 12:1877-1885, 1997.
37. Galway A.B., LaPolt P.S., Tsafriri A., Dargan C.M., Boime I., Hsueh A.J.: Recombinant follicle-stimulating hormone induces ovulation and tissue plasminogen activator expression in hypophysectomized rats. *Endocrinology*, 127:3023-3028, 1990.
38. Montgomery Rice V.C., Zusmanis K., Malter H., Mitchell-Leef D.: Pure FSH alone induces ovulation and subsequent pregnancy in the mouse resulting in fetal development. *Life Sci.*, 53:31-39, 1993.
39. Zelinski-Wooten M.B., Hutchison J.S., Hess D.L., Wolf D.P., Stouffer R.L.:

A bolus of recombinant human follicle stimulating hormone at midcycle induces periovulatory events following multiple follicular development in macaques. *Hum. Reprod.*, 13:554-560, 1998.
40. Zelinski-Wooten M.B., Lanzendorf S.E., Wolf D.P., Chandrasekher Y.A., Stouffer R.L.: Titrating luteinizing hormone surge requirements for ovulatory changes in primate follicles. I. Oocyte maturation and corpus luteum function. *J. Clin. Endocrinol. Metab.*, 73:577-583, 1991.
41. Chappel S.C., Howles C.: Reevaluation of the roles of luteinizing hormone and follicle-stimulating hormone in the ovulatory process. *Hum. Reprod.*, 6:1206-1012, 1991.
42. Shoham Z., Jacobs H.S., Insler V.: Luteinizing hormone: its role, mechanism of action, and detrimental effects when hypersecreted during the follicular phase. *Fertil. Steril.*, 59:1153-1161, 1993.
43. Thomas A., Ukamoto S., O'Shea F., MacLachlan V., Besanko M., Healy D.: Do raised serum luteinizing hormone levels during stimulation for in vitro fertilization predict outcome? *Br. J. Obstet. Gynaecol.*, 96:1328-1332, 1989.
44. Kovacs G.T., Baker H.W., Burger H.C., Lu J., Summerbell D.: Prognosis of pregnancies conceived by donor insemination with respect to the late follicular phase luteinizing hormone levels. *Br. J. Obstet. Gynaecol.*, 97:654-656, 1990.
45. Li T.C., Serle E., Warren M.A., Cooke I.D.: Is endometrial development in the peri-implantation period influenced by high concentrations of luteinizing hormone in the follicular phase? *Hum. Reprod.*, 8:1021-1024, 1993.

The Role of Luteinizing Hormone
in Folliculogenesis
and Ovulation Induction, pp. 53-68
Editor M. Filicori

Role of Estradiol in Oocyte Maturation and Fertilization

N.S. Macklon and B.C.J.M. Fauser

Division of Reproductive Medicine, Department of Obstetrics and Gynaecology
Erasmus University Medical Center Rotterdam (The Netherlands)

Abstract. *During the late-follicular phase of the normal menstrual cycle, serum follicle fluid estradiol concentrations are closely associated with dominant follicle development. Estrogens play important functional roles in the reproductive system by inducing the mid-cycle gonadotropin surge, and by stimulating endometrial proliferation and cervical mucus production. Follicle fluid estrogen concentrations have been shown to be correlated with outcome of* in vitro *fertilization.*

It has long been believed that increased estrogen levels are required for follicle (and oocyte) maturation. In fact, reduced estrogen output has long been held responsible for ovarian dysfunction in poycystic ovary syndrome. However, the use of human recombinant FSH in hypogonadotropic subjects has convincingly demonstrated that the two-cell, two gonadotropin concept is opertaive in the human. Minimal or absent theca cell androgen synthesis does not allow for sufficient substrate to be aromatized to estradiol under the influence of FSH. Surpringly, follicle development occurred up to the pre-ovulatory stage and was unaffected by low estrogen levels, suggesting that other factors infact drive growth of the follicle. Similar observations were made in patients incapable of producing estrogens due to steroid synthesis enzyme defects (chiefly due to mutations in the gene regulating cytochrome p450 C17 enzyme activity). Follicle growth could be stimulated, oocytes obtained and fertilized in vitro. *Recently, inactivating mutations of the LH receptor have been reported in women presenting with amenorrhea. However, multiple antral follicles were present despite low estrogen concentrations. This experiment of nature may provide additional information regrading the role of estrogens in oocyte quality and reproductive potential.*

A series of studies in the monkey has clearly shown that FSH alone is sufficient for oocyte maturation, fertilization and embryo development.

Human data regarding the presence of estrogen receptors (ER) or ER mRNA in oocytes, cumulus or granulosa cells are conflicting. Hopefully, the recently discovered estrogen receptor subtype (ERβ), predominantly expressed in the ovary, may help to further elucidate this matter. Certainly, in vitro experiments have shown that estrogens can influence oocyte quality. Non genomic effects of estrogens on human oocytes have also been reported.

Key words. Estradiol, oocyte, follicle, development, maturation.

Introduction

During the final stage of follicular development to the pre-ovulatory stage, when recruited follicles become FSH dependent[1], the oocyte undergoes important maturational processes. Within the dominant follicle, nuclear maturation of the oocyte involves the resumption of meiosis and its continuation up to metaphase II (MII). Maturation of the oocyte cytoplasm includes secretion of the zona pellucida, an extracellular matrix essential for binding sperm to the oocyte, and production of cortical granules which, following sperm-egg fusion, release proteases rendering the zona pellucida impenetrable to other sperm[2].

Serum and follicle estradiol concentrations are closely associated with dominant follicle development. Studies from our group have demonstrated a consistent relationship between estradiol production and follicular diameter > 9mm[3-5]. While it has long been believed that increased estrogen levels are required for follicle and oocyte maturation, recent data from *in vivo* and laboratory studies on humans and primates has called the role of oestradiol into question.

The two-cell two-gonadotropin concept

Estrogens play important functional roles in the reproductive system by inducing the mid-cycle gonadotropin surge, stimulating cervical mucus production and endometrial proliferation. Estradiol production is one of the principle functions of the developing follicle. During the FSH-dependent phase of follicular development, luteinizing hormone (LH) has a synergistic action with FSH. Theca cells are stimulated by LH to convert cholesterol into androstenedione (AD) and testosterone (T) by cytochrome p450 side chain cleavage oxidases and 3ß-hydroxy-steroid dehydrogenase. Aromatase activity in the granulosa cells is induced by FSH and converts AD and T into estrone and estradiol. In addition, FSH increases FSH receptor and induces LH receptor formation enabling LH to become a potent stimulator of aromatase activity during the late follicular phase[6,7]. The involvement of two cell types (granulosa and theca cells) and two hormones (LH and FSH) to produce estrogens from cholesterol has led to the concept of the 'two-cell, two-gonadotropin' theory. Laboratory derived evidence for this concept includes immunocytochemical studies and Northern blot analysis of RNA showing the cytochrome p450 C17 enzyme, responsible for conversion of progestins to androgens, to be restricted to the theca cell layer, consistent with the concept of theca cells as the major site for intra-ovarian androgen synthesis[8]. In addition, cytochrome p450 aromatase has been demonstrated in the granulosa cells of dominant follicles[9-11]. Evidence that this mechanism is operative *in-vivo* has come from animal and clinical studies. Using a rat model Mannaerts et al.[12] observed a three-fold increase in plasma estradiol when FSH was supplemented with a small amount of human chorionic gonadotropin (HCG). In 1971 Berger and Taymor[13] reported that an amenorrhoeic woman (due to pituitary irradiation) receiving human pituitary FSH alone showed no estradiol response and absent ovulation. In 1992 Schoot et al.[14] described the effects of recombinant FSH administration on a woman suffering from isolated gonadotropin deficiency due to previous hypophysectomy. This provided a unique model to assess the significance of LH for normal estradiol biosynthesis, since for the first time effects of FSH alone could be studied in the complete absence of endogenous and exogenous LH. Recombinant FSH (rec FSH) was administered daily by i.m. injections of one ampoule followed by two ampoules per day, which resulted in a clear rise in serum FSH concentrations from 1.2 to 8.5 IU/l. However, LH concentrations did not change with serum concentrations ranging between 0.09 and 0.38 IU/l. Serum estradiol concentrations showed a minimal but steady increase with maximal concentrations (236 pmol/l) still within the normal early follicular phase concentrations (Figure 1 and 2). The minimal increase in endometrial thickness observed suggested exposure to minimal amounts of estradiol.

This case provided conclusive evidence that the two-cell, two-gonadotropin concept is operative in the human. A subsequent study reported a normal increase in serum inhibin levels excluding the possibility of a granulosa cell defect per sé in these patients[15].

In-vitro Animal Studies

In-vitro animal studies have shown increased intra-follicular estradiol production to be mandatory for follicular growth. These studies have indicated that estradiol has a role in granulosa cell proliferation[16], enhancement of aromatase activity[17] and in increasing expression of FSH receptors and induction of LH receptors in granulosa cells[18,19]. A regulatory role for estradiol on

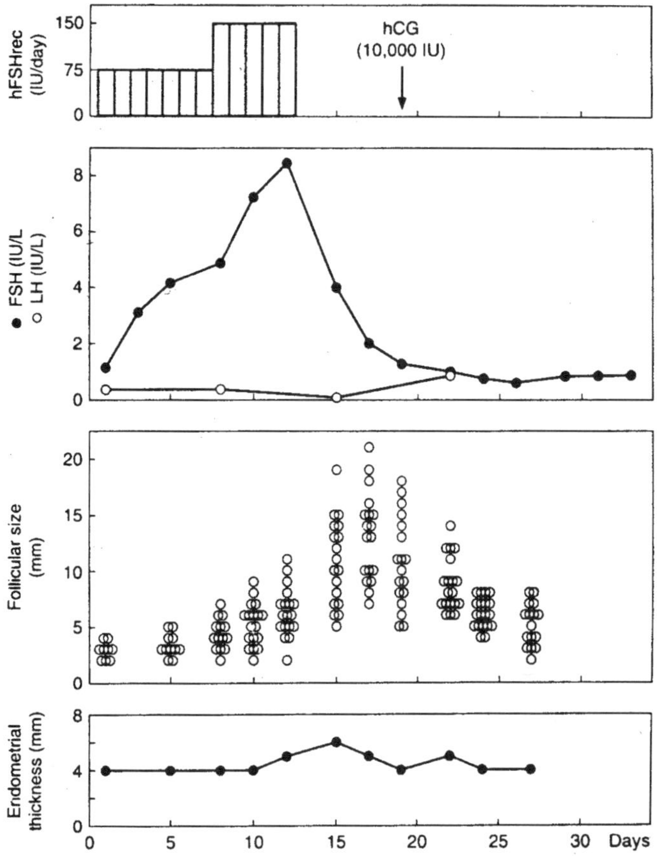

FIGURE 1 - *Endocrine and sonographic observations in a single patient with isolated gonadotropin deficiency receiving daily injections of rec FSH. Serum FSH and LH levels, follicle diameter and endometrial thickness are shown. HCG, Human chorionic gonadotropin.* (Reproduced with permission from B.C. Schoot et al.[14], The Endocrine Society).

androgen production by theca cells, possibly by an inhibitory action on cyto chrome p450 C17 activity in the theca cells has also been reported[20]. Estrogens play an important role in the enhancement of antrum formation[21] and of intercellular gap junction formation[22] and estradiol may also have a role in inhibiting apoptotic changes in ovarian follicles[23].

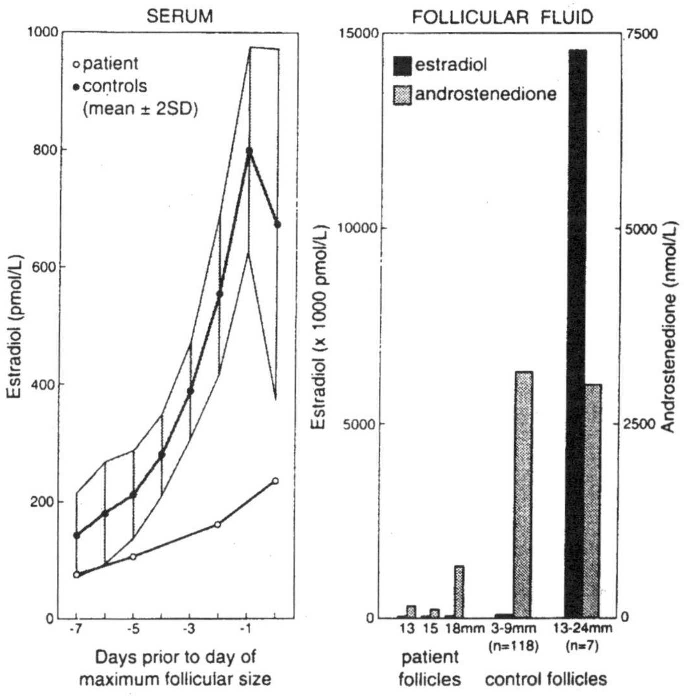

FIGURE 2 - *Serum estradiol levels and follicle fluid estradiol and androstenedione concentrations (three follicles, 13-18 mm in diameter) from the patient referred to in Figure 1 during treatment with rec FSH are shown, together with those determined in regularly cycling control subjects.* (Reproduced with permission from B.C. Schoot et al.[14], The Endocrine Society).

In-vitro Primate and Human Studies

In-vitro studies of the effects of exogenous estrogens on granulosa cells have elucidated important differences between laboratory animals and primates. In rats, estradiol plays a critically important role in the proliferation of granulosa cells[24] but this does not appear to be the case in the primate since primate granulosa cells do not contain estradiol receptors[25]. Similarly, while in the rat, exogenous estrogens stimulate granulosa cell steroidogenesis[17], this does not occur in primates. However, Iwai[26] was able to demonstrate estrogen receptors in human granulosa cells, but only in those from mature, preovulatory follicles; not in pre-antral follicles. These findings may point to a stage and cell specific action for estradiol.

Support for autocrine roles for steroids in modulating the maturational processes required before fertilization can occur has come from the recent detection of messenger RNA for ER in human oocytes[27] combined with the localization of androgen receptors in macaque oocytes[28]. 17 α-hydroxylase activity[29] and 3ß-HSD activity[30] has also been identified in human oocytes. However, the action of FSH on the maturing follicle and oocyte would appear not to be mediated by estradiol but by non-steroidal mediators such as IGF, inhibin and activin[31,32]. In an *in-vitro* study of rhesus monkey oocyte maturation, addition of inhibin and activin were found to accelerate progession to meiosis II and the germinal vesicle[33]. Moreover, exposure to medium containing inhibin and activin significantly increased the percentage of MII oocytes that fertilized compared with control oocytes (68% versus 25% respectively).

Clinical Models and *in-vivo* Primate Studies

Support for an important role for estradiol in follicular maturation has been provided by studies which demonstrate a correlation between follicular estradiol production, follicular fluid content and the health of the follicle[34,35]. However, recent case studies indicate that this correlation may reflect estradiol acting as marker for oocyte maturation rather than as a factor controlling maturation. In the case report referred to earlier[14] where rec FSH was administered to a woman with isolated gonadotropin deficiency, the observed minimal increase in endometrial thickness in response to treatment suggested exposure to minimal amounts of estradiol. Despite low estradiol synthesis, multiple follicles increased in size up to a diameter of 22mm in this woman. Three follicles were punctured, revealing intrafollicular estradiol concentrations 1000-fold lower than that found in follicles of similar size under normal conditions. However, the low estradiol levels present did not compromise follicle growth.

Possible sources for the residual estradiol activity observed in this patient include the conversion of adrenal androgens[36], low level constitutive androgen production by the theca cells or stimulated androgen production by locally produced growth factors. Similar observations were subsequently reported in two[37] and seven[38] hypogonadotropic women. Oocyte quality was not assessed in these studies.

Describing a further model for investigating the role of estrogens in follicular development, Rabinovici et al.[39] reported studies carried out on a 30 year old woman with a severe form of 17α hydroxylase deficiency. After receiving gonadotropin releasing hormone (GnRH) agonist to suppress endogenous

LH and FSH secretion, the patient was treated with a follicular recruitment protocol consisting of purified urinary FSH. Several follicles developed under this regimen and the patient was given human chorionic gonadotropin (hCG) and the follicles aspirated. The follicular growth occurred in the absence of a significant rise in estradiol in the peripheral blood (<74 pmol/l). Moreover, follicular fluid levels of testosterone (<0.03 nmol/l compared to 44-180 nmol/l in control follicular fluid) and estradiol (<1 nmol/l compared to 1,330-7,200 nmol/l in control follicular fluid) determined by radioimunoassay were barely detectable. Following *in-vitro* fertilization of the aspirated oocytes, two developed to the 7-cell stage but no pregnancy was achieved.

Some abnormalities in the steroidogenic activity of the granulosa cells collected from this patient were observed. The authors reported an increased capacity of the granulosa cells to produce progesterone and a reduced ability of the granulosa cells to aromatize exogenous androgen.

These differences may have been due to the estradiol deficiency in the follicular environment.

Reporting a woman with a partial 17,20 desmolase deficiency causing very low androgen and estrogen production, Pellicer et al.[40] found administration of FSH to result in multiple follicular development. Only 11 of the 19 oocytes obtained fertilized, and despite the transfer of four embryos, no pregnancy ensued. The endometrial response to a low estradiol milieu may have been a factor mitigating against pregnancy in these two cases. While reports of pregancies and births are lacking in women with defective 17-hydroxylase enzyme activity, the occurence of ovarian hyperstimulation syndrome despite very low estradiol levels in a cytochrome p450 C17 deficient patient has recently been reported[41].

More recently, two female patients have been described with inactivating mutations of the LH receptor. In one, ovarian morphology was normal with multiple antral follicles[42]. Serum FSH and LH concentrations were elevated. However serum estradiol levels were low and could not be augmented by the administration of hCG. Despite absent theca cell stimulation and low estrogen concentrations, multiple antral follicles were present. In another woman presenting with amenorrhea and normal development of secondary sex characteristics, serum estrogen levels remained in the range normally seen during the early follicular phase of the menstrual cycle, sufficient to allow for normal pubertal feminization[43]. The ovaries were enlarged with multiple large cysts. In addition to providing further evidence that estrogens are not required for follicle development, these subjects confirm the two-cell-two gonadotropin concept.

Mutations in the CYP19 gene (localized on on chromosome 15,q21.1 region) which results in total absence of aromataze enzyme activity have recently been described in two unrelated women[44,45]. Large ovarian cysts were described in both patients, suggesting that growth of antral follicles can occur in the absence of intra-ovarian estrogen biosynthesis.

These studies demonstrate that a high local estradiol (or testosterone) level is not required for follicular growth and development in women. However, low levels of estradiols may be important for follicular function, as suggested by some of the alterations in granulosa cell steroidogenesis observed in cells collected form the patient with 17α hydroxylase deficiency.

Recent studies in primates have suggested that the maturational role of estradiol may be of greater importance in the latter stages of oocyte development and preparing the mature oocyte for fertilization. In a study of rhesus monkeys who had received an 3ß-HSD inhibitor, Zelinski-Wooten et al.[46] showed that despite estradiol suppression to 7% of that of controls, follicular growth and oocyte nuclear maturity were unaltered. However, the fertilisability of metaphase II oocytes was just 15% in the study group, as compared with 65% in the control group. Evaluating the developmental potential of GnRH antagonist-treated macaque embryos given recFSH alone or in combination with recLH, Weston et al.[47] showed a similar ability for fertilised oocytes in both groups to develop to hatched blastocysts with a definitive inner cell mass. However, a significant difference was seen in cryosurvival (56% versus 78%) and in developmental rate to the hatched blastocyst (12 versus 10 days) between embryos from the rec FSH alone and the combination group respectively. This data provides further evidence that FSH alone during the pre-ovulatory interval is adequate for the gametogenic events required to produce embryos that develop either *in-vitro* or *in-vivo*; however exposure to LH, and hence estradiol may improve embryo viability and the rate of development.

Human IVF Studies

Human IVF studies have considered the role of LH and estradiol response to follicle-stimulating hormone on IVF outcome. Using data from 3 studies, Loumaye et al.[48] showed that serum levels of estradiol obtained on the day of hCG administration correlated positively with the number of oocytes retrieved and inversely with the fertilization rate. A wide range of estradiol-oocyte ratios were detected among the subjects and an 'optimal' estradiol-oocyte ratio above and below which live birth rates fell was identified. While a pregnancy rate of 5.3% per oocyte pick-up was observed in those with an estradiol-oocyte ratio of <70 pg estradiol/ml per oocyte, and a rate of 18-24% was observed in those with a ratio of > 140 pg/ml per oocyte, a significantly higher pregnancy rate of 31% per oocyte pick up was seen in those women with an intermediate estradiol-oocyte ratio between 70 and 140 pg/ml. There was, however no difference between the groups in the total number of developing follicles or fertilization rates. A high estradiol-oocyte ratio may affect pregnancy rates by reducing endometrial receptivity[49]. Conversely, too low a ratio may indicate a suboptimal LH level, as occurs in hypogonadotropic hypogonadism where poor quality oocytes are obtained, thus suggesting a mediating role for estradiol in oocyte maturation. In Loumaye's study, LH levels measured after down-regulation with a GnRH agonist did not correlate with the number of oocytes retrieved or the oocyte fertilization rate. The lack of a simple LH value to predict responses may reflect the very low LH levels required to influence estradiol synthesis[49]. In a recent prospective study[50] of normal women undergoing GnRH agonist down regulation prior IVF treatment, profound LH suppression to levels at or below the limits of assay sensitivity (≤0.5 IU/l) was associated with a reduced cohort of embryos and a reduced estradiol-oocyte ratio. However, the developmental capacity of those embryos remaining after selection for transfer was unaffected by the degree of LH suppression.

Further data from human IVF studies have shown that the ratio of estrogens to androgens in the follicular fluid correlates with oocyte fertilization and cleavage. In a study of 28 women undergoing an IVF treatment cycle, Yding Anderson[51] analysed follicular fluid from 14 women who subsequently became pregnant and 14 who did not conceive. While no difference was observed between pregnancy-assocated follicles and follicles not associated with pregnancy with respect to free and total estradiol or T concentrations, pregnancy was associated with those follicles which showed a significantly higher estradiol/T ratio than follicles from which the oocyte failed to implant or did not cleave *in-vitro*. This study confirmed an earlier report[52] suggesting a correlation between the estradiol ratio/androgen ratio and ability of the oocyte to fertilize and implant. A reduction in estradiol/androgen ratio may reflect or indeed underlie early follicular atresia from which the oocyte can be 'rescued' if sufficent estradiol is supplemented.

Novel Estradiol Actions and Receptors

Recently, non-genomic effects of estradiol have been reported which may shed some light on the function of estradiol in preparing the pre-ovulatory oocyte for fertilization. Non-genomic mechanisms of steroid activity are those which do not involve a modification of gene activity. Tesarik and Mendoza[53] have demonstrated that a membrane-impermeant oestradiol conjugate exerts a direct nongenomic effect on maturing human oocytes by inducing a series of transient increases in the intracellular free calcium concentration. Characterizing the pattern of these increases in intracellular calcium, they showed that while the initial increase was due to influx of extracellular calcium ions, a subsequent series of oscillations in intracellular calcium concentration originated from release of intra-cellular calcium stores. While such oscillations of intracellular calcium may occur spontaneously in murine oocytes, an estadiol stimulus appears to be required in the human oocyte.

Following the observation that the exposure of oocytes to the membrane-impermeable oestradiol conjugate during *in-vitro* maturation improved fertilization and the post-fertilization potential without any obvious effects on nuclear maturation, Tesarik and Mendoza[53] suggested that oestradiol may indeed influence cytoplasmic maturation by acting at the oocyte surface. In subsequent work they were able to demonstrate an antogonistic effect of androstenedione on the calcium oscillation inducing effects of estradiol. If oscillations in intra-cellular calcium concentrations represent an important maturational process, then their prevention by in-vivo exposure to low estrogen/androgen ratios would be consistent with the impaired development potential shown by oocytes exposed to reduced estradiol/androgen ratios in the follicular fluid. Moreover, a crucial role for the ratio of estradiol to androgens rather than their absolute levels in the follicular fluid would explain the ability of oocytes from a woman with 17α-hydroxylase deficiency to undergo fertilization[39]. When intrafollicular concentrations of androgens are low, relatively low concentrations of estrogens may still be sufficent to allow normal cytoplasmic maturation. Although the functional significance of intracellular calcium oscillations in the maturing human oocyte remains unclear, they have been shown to represent an early reaction of oocytes to the fertilizing spermatazoon[54] and may therefore play a facilitatory role, indicating a degree of oocyte 'capacitation'.

Human data regarding the presence of estrogen receptors or estrogen receptor (ER) mRNA in oocytes, cumulus or granulosa cells are conflicting. The recent discovery of an estrogen receptor subtype, ERß[55] which in the human is predominantly expressed in the ovary[56] may help to further elucidate this matter. Calculations of the ratio between the ERα and ERß mRNA have shown that in human granulosa cells, only the newly isolated ERß subtype is expressed[56]. Throughout the rest of the ovary, the amounts of ERα and ERß mRNA appear to be approximately equal. The presence of ERß receptor in human granulosa cells suggests that it is likely to play an important role in the regulation of follicular growth and oocyte development.

Conclusions

In contrast to what was previously believed, it has now been demonstrated that increased oestradiol biosynthesis is not required for follicle growth in the human. The growth of the follicle may be driven by other as yet unidentified non-steroidal intra-ovarian factors.

The role of oestradiol in determining human oocyte quality remains uncertain.

The discovery of novel mechanisms of estradiol action, previously unidentified receptor subtypes, and the reports of naturally occuring clinical 'models' such as those outlined in this article should lead to a greater understanding of the role of estradiol in follicular and oocyte maturation.

References

1. Fauser B.C.J.M., Van Heusden A.M.: Manipulation of human ovarian function: physiological concepts and clinical consequences. *Endocrine Rev.*, 18:71-106, 1997.
2. Dean J.: Biology of mammalian fertilization: role of the zona pellucida. *J. Clin. Invest.*, 89:1055-1059, 1992.
3. Pache T.D., Hop W.C., de Jong F.H., Leerentveld R.A., van Geldrop H., van de Kamp T.M., Gooren L.J., Fauser B.C.J.M.: 17 beta-oestradiol, androstenedione and inhibin levels in fluid from individual follicles of normal and polycystic ovaries, and in ovaries from androgen treated female to male transsexuals. *Clin. Endocrinol.* (Oxf), 36:565-571, 1992.
4. Van Dessel H.J.H.M., Schipper I., Pache T.D., van Geldrop H., de Jong F.H., Hop W.C., Fauser B.C.J.M.: Normal human follicle development: and evaluation of correlations with oestradiol, androstenedione and progesterone levels in individual follicles. *Clin. Endocrinol.* (Oxf), 44:191-198, 1996
5. Van Santbrink E.J.P., Hop W.C., van Dessel H.J.H.M., de Jong F.H., Fauser B.C.J.M.: Decremental follicle-stimulating hormone and dominant follicle development during the normal menstrual cycle. *Fertil. Steril.*, 64:37-43, 1995.
6. Hillier S., Reichart L.E., van Hall E.V.: Control of preovulatory follicular estrogen biosynthesis in the human ovary. *J. Clin. Endocrinol. Metab.*, 52, 847-856, 1981.
7. Hsueh A.J., Bicsak T.A., Jia X.C., Dahl K.D., Fauser B.C., Galway A.B., Czekela N., Pavlou S.N., Papkoff H., Keene J.: Granulosa cells as hormone targets: the role of biologically active follicle-stimulating hormone in reproduction. *Recent Preg. Horm. Res.*, 45-209-273, 1989.
8. Tonetta S.A., di Zerega G.S.: Intragonadal regulation of follicular matura-

tion. *Endocr. Rev.*, 10:205-229,1989.

9. Sasano H., Okamato M., Mason J.I., Simpsin E.R., Mendelson C.R., Sasano N., Silverberg S.G.: Immunolocalization of aromataze, 17α-hydroxylase and side schain cleavage cyctochrome P450 in the human ovary. *J. Reprod. Fertil.*, 85:163-169, 1989.
10. Doody K.J., Lorence M.C., Mason J.I., Simpson E.R.: Expression of mRNA species encoding steroidogenic enzymes in human follicles and corpora lutea throughout the menstrual cycle. *J. Clin. Endocrinol. Metab.*, 70:1041-1045, 1990.
11. Suzuki T., Sasano H., Tamura M., Aoki M., Fukaya T., Yajima A., Nagura H., Mason J.I.: Temporal and spatial localization of steroidogenic enzymes in premenopausal human ovaries: *in situ* hybridization and immunohistochemical study. *Mol. Cell Endocrinol. Metab.*, 97:135-143,1993.
12. Mannaerts B., De Leeuw R., Geelen J., Van Ravenstein A., Van Wezenbeek P., Schuurs A., Kloosterboer H.: Comparative *in vitro* and *in vivo* studies on the biological characteristics of recombinant human FSH. *Endocrinology*, 129:2623-2630, 1991.
13. Berger M.J., Taymor M.L.: The role of luteinizing hormone in human follicular maturation and function. *Am. J. Obstet. Gynecol.*, 111:708-712, 1971.
14. Schoot D.C., Coelingh Bennink, Mannaerts B.M., Lamberts S.W., Bouchard P., Fauser B.C.: Human recombinant follicle-stimulating hormone induces growth of preovulatory follicles without concomitant increase in androgen and estrogen biosynthesis in a woman with isolated gonadotrophin deficiency. *J. Clin. Endocrinol. Metab.*, 74:1471-1473,1992.
15. Schoot D.C., Harlin J., Shoham Z., Mannaerts B.M., Lahlou N., Bouchard P., Bennink H.J., Fauser B.C.: Recombinant human follicle-stimulating hormone and ovarian response in gonadotrophin-deficient women. *Hum. Reprod.*, 9:1237-1242, 1994.
16. Rao M.C., Midgley A.R. Jr, Richards J.S.: Hormonal regulation of ovarian cellular proliferation. *Cell*, 14:71-78, 1978.
17. Adashi E.Y., Hsueh A.J.W.: Estrogens augment the stimulation of ovarian aromatase activity by follicle-stimulating hormone in cultures rat granulosa cells. *J. Biol. Chem.*, 257:6077-6083, 1982
18. Louvet J.P., Vaitukaitis J.L.: Induction of follicle-stimulating hormone (FSH) receptors in rat ovaries by estrogen priming. *Endocrinology*, 99:758-63, 1976.
19. Richards J.S., Jonassen J.A., Rolfes A.I., Kersey K., Reichert L.E. Jr.: Adenosine-3'5'-monophosphate, luteinizing hormone receptor and progesterone during granulosa cell differentiation: effects of estradiol and follicle-

stimulating hormone. *Endocrinology*, 104:765-771, 1979.
20. Erickson G.F., Magoffin D.A., Dyer C.A., Hofeditz C.: The ovarian androgen producing cells: a review of structure/function relationships. *Endocrine Rev.*, 6:371-399, 1985.
21. Richards J.S., Jongssen J.A., Kersey K.A.: Evidence that changes in tonic luteinizing hormone secretion determine the growth of preovulatory follicles in the rat. *Endocrinology*, 107:641-648, 1980
22. Merk F.B., Botticelli C.R., Albright J.T.: An intercellular response to estrogen by granulosa cells in the rat ovary; an electron microscope study. *Endocrinology*, 90:992-1007, 1972.
23. Billig H., Furata I., Hsueh A.J.W.: Estrogens inhibit and androgens enhance ovarian granulosa cell apoptosis. *Endocrinology*, 133:2204-2212, 1993.
24. Richards J.S.: Estradiol receptor content in rat granulosa cells during follicular development: modification of estradiol and gonadotropins. *Endocrinology*, 97:1174-1184, 1975.
25. Hild-Petito S., Stouffer R.L., Brenner R.M.: Immunocytochemical localization of estradiol and progesterone receptors in the monkey throughout the menstrual cycle. *Endocrinology*, 123:2896-2905,1988.
26. Iwai T., Nanbu Y., Iwai M., Taii S., Fujii S., Mori M.: Immunohistochemical localization of estrogen receptors and progesterone receptors in the human ovary throughout the mesntrual cycle. *Virchows Arch.*, 417:369-378, 1990.
27. Wu T.-C.J., Wang L., Wan Y.-J.Y.: Detection of estrogen receptor messenger ribonucleic acid in human oocytes and cumulus-oocyte complexes using reverse transcriptase-polymerase chain reaction. *Fertil. Steril.*, 59:54-59, 1993.
28. Hild-Petito S., West N.B., Brenner R.M., Stouffer R.L.: Localization of androgen receptor in the follicle and corpus luteum of the primate ovary during the menstrual cycle. *Biol Reprod.*, 44:561-568, 1991.
29. Tamura T., Kitawaki J., Yamomoto T., Osawa Y., Kominami S., Takemori S.: Immunohistochemical localization of 17(-hydroxylase/C17-20 lyase and aromatase cytochrome P-450 in the human ovary during the menstrual cycle. *J. Endocrinol.*, 135:589-595, 1992.
30. Suzuki S., Endo Y., Fujiwara T., Tanaka S., Iizuka R.: Cytochemical study of steroid-producing activities of human oocytes. *Fertil. Steril.*, 39:682-689, 1983.
31. Miro F., Hillier S.G.: Relative effects of inhibin and activin on steroid hormone synthesis in primate granulosa cells. *J. Clin. Endocrinol. Metab.*, 75:1556-1561, 1992.
32. Findlay J.K.: Peripheral and local regulators of folliculogenesis. *Reprod.*

Fertil. Dev., 6:127-139, 1994.

33. Alak B.M., Smith G.D., Woodruff T.K., Stouffer R.L., Wolf D.P.: Enhancement of primate ooctye maturation and fertilization in vitro by inhibin A and activin A. *Fertil. Steril.*, 66:646-653, 1996.
34. McNatty K.P.: Hormonal correlates of follicular development in the human ovary. *Aust. J. Biol. Sci.*, 34:249-268, 1981.
35. Tonetta S.A., diZerega G.S.: Intragonadal regulation of follicular maturation. *Endocrine Rev.*, 10:205-229, 1989.
36. Ben-Chetrit A., Gotlieb L., Wong P.Y., Casper R.F.: Ovarian response to recombinant human follicle-stimulating hormone in luteinizing hormone-depleted women: examination of the two cell, two gonadotrophin theory. *Fertil. Steril.*, 65:711-717, 1996.
37. Shoham Z., Mannaerts B., Insler V., Coelingh-Bennink H.: Induction of follicular growth using recombinant human follicle-stimulaing hormone in two volounteer women with hypogonadotropic hypogonadism. *Fertil. Steril.*, 59:738-742, 1993.
38. Schoot D.C., Harlin J., Shoham Z., Mannaerts B.M., Lahlou N., Bouchard P., Bennink H.J., Fauser B.C.: Recombinant human follicle-stimulating hormone and ovarian reponse in gonadotrophin-deficient women. *Hum. Reprod.*, 9:1237-1242, 1994.
39. Rabinovici J., Blankstein J., Goldman B., Rudak E., Dor Y., Pariente C., Geier A., Lunenfeld B., Mashiach S.: *In vitro* fertilization and primary embryonic cleavage are possible in 17α-hydroxylase deficiency despite extremely low intrafollicular 17ß-estradiol. *J. Clin. Endocrinol. Metab.*, 68:693-697, 1989.
40. Pellicer A., Miro F., Sampaio M., Gomez E., Bonilla-Musoles F.M.: In vitro fertilization as a diagnostic and therapeutic tool in a patient with partial 17,20-desmolase deficiency. *Fertil. Steril.*, 55:970-975, 1991.
41. Meirow D., Schenker J.G., Rosler A.: Ovarian hyperstimulation syndrome with low oestradiol in non-classical 17α-hydroxylase, 17,20-lyase deficieny: what is the role of oestrogens? *Hum. Reprod.*, 11:2119-2121, 1996.
42. Toledo S.P., Brunner H.G., Kraaij H., Post M., Dahia P.L., Hayashida C.Y., Kremer H., Themmen A.P.: An inactivating mutation of the luteinizing hormone receptor causes amenorrhea in a 46,XX female. *J. Clin. Endocrinol. Metab.*, 81:3850-3854, 1996.
43. Latronico A.C., Anasti J., Arnhold I.J., Rapaport R., Mendonca B.B., Bloise W., Casczo M., Tsigos C., Chrousos G.P.: Testicular and ovarian resistance to luteinizing hormone caused by inactivating mutations of the luteinizing hormone-receptor gene. *N. Engl. J. Med.*, 334:507-512, 1996.
44. Conte F.A., Grumbach M.M., Ito Y., Fisher C.R., Simpson E.R.: A syndrome

of female pseudohermaphroditism, hypergonadotropic hypogonadism, and multicystic ovaries assocaited with missense mutations in the gene encoding aromatase (P450arom). *J. Clin. Endocrinol. Metab.*, 78:1287-1292, 1994.

45. Morishima A., Grumbach M.M., Simpson E.R., Fisher C., Qin K.: Aromatase deficiency in male and female siblings caused by a novel mutation and the physiological role of estrogens. *J. Clin. Endocrinol. Metab.*, 80:3689-3698, 1995.
46. Zelinski-Wooten M.B., Hess D.L., Wolf D.P., Stouffer R.L.: Steroid reduction during ovarian stimulation impairs oocyte fertilization, but not folliculogenesis, in rhesus monkeys. *Fertil. Steril.*, 61:1147-1155, 1994.
47. Weston A.M., Zelinski-Wooten M.B., Hutchison J.S., Stouffer R.L., Wolf D.P.: Developmental potential of embryos produced by in-vitro fertilization from gonadotrophin-releasing hormone antagonist-treated macaques stimulated with recombinant human follicle stimulating hormone alone or in combination with lutienizing hormone. *Hum. Reprod.*, 11:608-613, 1996.
48. Loumaye E., Engrand P., Howles C.M., O'Dea L.: Assessment of the role of serum luteinizing hormone and estradiol response to follicle-stimulating hormone on in vitro fertilization treatment outcome. *Fertil. Steril.*, 67:889-899, 1997.
49. Chappel S.C., Howles C.: Reevaluation of the roles of luteinizing hormone and follicle-stimulating hormone in the ovulatory process. *Hum. Reprod.*, 6:1206-1212,1991.
50. Fleming R., Lloyd F., Herbert M., Fenwick J., Griffiths T., Murdoch A.: Effects of profound suppression of luteinizing hormone during ovarian stimulation on follicular activity, oocyte and embryo function in cycles stimulated with purified follicle stimulating hormone. *Hum. Reprod.*, 13:1788-1792, 1998.
51. Yding Anderson C.: Characteristics of human follicular fluid associated with successful conception after in vitro fertilization. *J. Clin. Endocrinol. Metab.*, 77:1227-1234, 1993.
52. Chabab A., Hedon B., Arnal F., Diafouka F., Bressot N., Flandre O., Cristol P.: Follicular steroids in relation to oocyte development and human ovarian stimulation protocols. *Hum. Reprod.*, 1:449-454, 1986.
53. Tesarik J., Mendoza C.: Nongenomic effects of 17(-estradiol on maturing human oocytes: relationship to oocyte developmental potential. *J. Clin. Endocrinol. Metab.*, 80:1438-1443, 1995.
54. Taylor C.T., Lawrence Y.M., Kingsland C.R., Biljan M.M., Cuthbertson K.S.R.: Oscillations in intracellular free calcium induced by spermatozoa in human oocytes at fertilization. *Hum. Reprod.*, 8:2174-2179, 1993.

55. Kuiper G., Enmark E., Pelto-Huikko M., Nilsson S., Gustafsson J.: Cloning of a novel estrogen receptor expressed in rat prostate and ovary. *Proc. Natl. Acad. Sci. USA.*, 93:5925-5930, 1996.
56. Enmark E., Pelto-Huikko M., Grandien K., Lagercrantz S., Lagerkrantz J., Fried G., Nordenskjöld M., Gustafsson J.: Human estrogen receptor (-gene structure, chromasomal localization, and expression pattern. *J. Clin. Endocrinol. Metab.*, 82:4258-4265,1997.

The Role of Luteinizing Hormone
in Folliculogenesis
and Ovulation Induction, pp. 69-78
Editor M. Filicori

Roles of Androgens in Ovarian Folliculogenesis

S.G. Hillier

Reproductive Medicine Laboratory, Department of Obstetrics and Gynaecology
University of Edinburgh Centre for Reproductive Biology
Edinburgh (United Kingdom)

Abstract. *Androgens are synthesized in ovarian follicles where they serve both as oestrogen precursors and paracrine regulators of granulosa cell function. This chapter examines the evidence that the granulosa cell androgen receptor system is developmentally regulated and concludes that this may explain why both stimulatory (tropic) and inhibitory (atretic) effects have been ascribed to follicular androgens.*

Key words. Gonadotropins, ovulation, atresia, growth factors, receptors, intracellular signalling.

Introduction

The normal production of sex hormones and gametes in women depends on appropriate stimulation of the gonads by adequate amounts of the pituitary gonadotrophins follicle-stimulating hormone (FSH) and luteinising hormone (LH). However, ovarian function is also critically dependent on the local production of paracrine factors that mediate and modulate the actions of FSH and LH[1]. In this lecture I briefly sketch the concept of paracrine gonadal control, highlighting roles played by locally produced androgen and androgen receptors.

Gonadotropic Control of Folliculogenesis

Follicular growth in the ovaries is mainly driven by FSH, acting directly on granulosa cells. Granulosa cells express FSH receptors from the time they are morphologically recognisable, and FSH acting via cyclic AMP mediated post-receptor signalling regulates the genes that orchestrate the proliferation and differentiation of these cells in the growing follicle. LH is also necessary for normal follicular growth, acting on surrounding thecal cells to promote the formation of androgens that are consumed by granulosa cells in the formation of oestrogens during late preovulatory development[2]. Granulosa cells express androgen receptors throughout most of the life-cycle of the follicle, and androgen appears to serve an important function in modulating the growth and differentiating functions of FSH on these cells[3]. A consequence of FSH action on granulosa cells is the increased expression of genes encoding inhibin, which reciprocally modulates LH-stimulated androgen formation in the theca[4]. This paracrine feedback loop is believed to underpin the endocrine regulation of ovarian follicular development and oestrogen secretion. Evidence for the crucial role played by androgen will now be reviewed.

Androgen Secretion

The ovaries are major sites of androgen production and metabolism - every molecule of oestrogen they synthesise is derived from a molecule of androgen[5]. Androstenedione and to a much lesser extent testosterone are synthesised by ovarian follicles throughout their most active phase of antral growth. During the follicular phase of the human menstrual cycle, the ovary contributes about 30 percent of the total blood androstenedione. The adrenal accounts for the rest, as revealed by the decline in circulating androstenedione levels that occurs in response to adrenal suppression with dexamethasone[6]. At mid-cycle the ovarian contribution arises to about 60 percent due to the increased synthesis and secretion of the steroid in the preovulatory follicle (see above)[7]. The ovary also secretes small amounts of testosterone but most of the testosterone in blood is derived from peripheral metabolism of androstenedione.

With age, follicle numbers in the ovaries gradually decline until the menopause is reached, when ovulation ceases. Once devoid of preovulatory follicles or corpora lutea, the ovaries cease oestrogen synthesis, and blood levels of oestrogen decline. However, post-menopausal ovaries continue to secrete androstenedione and small amounts of testosterone synthesised in secondary interstitial tissue. Occasionally, there is evidence of stromal hyperplasia and ovarian androgen secretion associated with circulating testosterone levels in the male range, which results in hirsutism and virilisation. It is assumed that the low blood oestrogen levels present in post-menopausal women are mainly derived from the extra-glandular conversion of adrenal androstenedione, since castration of postmenopausal women does not reduce oestrogen levels whereas adrenalectomy following castration does[6]. However, long-term suppression of pituitary gonadotropin secretion in postmenopausal women by treatment with a LHRH agonist causes a significant reduction in circulating testosterone and oestradiol levels, indicating a continued dependence of ovarian androgen secretion on gonadotropic stimulation after the menopause[8].

Oestrogen Secretion

The onset of follicular oestrogen secretion reflects a functional interplay between the two major steroidogenic cell types in the follicle – granulosa and thecal – regulated by FSH and LH. LH stimulates precursor androgen synthesis in the theca and FSH stimulates granulosa cell aromatase activity. Thus both cell types and both gonadotropins are crucial to oestrogen synthesis[49-11].

By the mid-follicular phase, the dominant follicle is recognisable as the largest healthy follicle in either ovary[12]. At this time, maintenance of its status as the dominant follicle becomes increasingly dependent on LH. As discussed above, LH receptors are constitutively present on thecal cells and develop on granulosa cells following stimulation by FSH. Thus the dominant follicle secretes increased amounts of androstenedione as well as oestradiol in response to stimulation by LH[13]. Paracrine signalling (granulosa on theca) is thought to contribute to the selective enhancement of LH-responsive androgen synthesis that occurs in this follicle[14-16]. In vitro, LH co-ordinately stimulates aromatase activity and inhibin synthesis in granulosa cells from the dominant follicle[17], and inhibin potentially enhances LH-stimulated thecal androgen synthesis[18]. Thus inhibin is thought likely to participate in the paracrine system that leads to enhanced secretion of oestrogen by the dominant follicle.

Paracrine Regulation

Locally produced steroidal and non-steroidal factors modulate gonadotropin action on ovarian cells, thereby influencing the sensitivity of maturing follicles to FSH and LH[1]. Intrafollicular factors in this category include the insulin-like growth factors (IGFs)[19] pro-inflammatory cytokines[20] epidermal growth factor (EGF)/transforming growth factor-α (TGF-α)[21] and members of the TGF-ß superfamily of growth/differentiation factors[22] that includes inhibin[4], activin[23,24] and germ-cell derived factor (GDF-9)[25]. Also implicated are kit ligand/Stem Cell Factor and hepatocyte growth factor (HGF)[26].

As discussed above, inhibin is likely to be of particular relevance to the ovarian paracrine system, since its formation is under FSH control in granulosa cells of the developing follicle. Not only is inhibin a major endocrine secretion of the ovary that participates, with oestradiol, in negative feedback regulation of pituitary FSH secretion[27] but it locally augments LH-stimulated thecal androgen synthesis[4]. Conversely, theca-derived androgen not only exerts reciprocal paracrine regulation of granulosa cell function[28] but is also the essential substrate for oestrogen synthesis.

Paracrine Androgen Action

A major influence on granulosa cell function, including inhibin formation, is exerted by androgens produced by LH-stimulated theca cells[29,30]. In rat ovary, granulosa cell androgen receptors bind androgen[31,32] and modulate cAMP-responsive gene expression[33,34]. Granulosa cell androgen receptor mRNA and protein are down-regulated during FSH-induced preovulatory follicular development, suggesting that paracrine androgen action might be influenced by development-related changes in androgen receptor expression[35,36].

To determine the location and developmental regulation of androgen receptors in primate ovary, we used quantitative immunocytochemistry to assess androgen receptor distribution in relation to preovulatory follicular development in the common marmoset (*Callithrix jacchus*), a New World primate that ovulates 2-4 follicles in each ~28-day ovarian cycle[37]. Specific androgen receptor immunostaining occurred mainly in granulosa cell nuclei, with little or no specific staining in theca, stroma or oocytes. Granulosa cell androgen receptor immunostaining was most abundant in healthy preantral/early antral follicles, being low or absent from preovulatory follicles and corpora lutea. Diffeences in granulosa cell androgen receptor immunostaining between immature (0.1-1.0 mm diameter) and preovulatory (2.0 mm diameter) follicles were quantified using videodensitometry, and the average androgen receptor level in granulosa cells of nonovulatory follicles proved to be 4.2 times higher than that in granulosa cells of preovulatory follicles.

The relatively high abundance of androgen receptors in the granulosa cells of immature follicles presumably has physiological relevance. Locally produced steroidal and nonsteroidal factors, including androgens, are thought to promote the FSH responsiveness of immatur follicules, thereby contributing to the mechanism determining which follicles are 'selected' to achieve full preovulatory maturity[3].

The functional relevance of androgen receptor loss in preovulatory follicles is unknown. However, in vitro studies on marmoset granulosa cell cultures have shown that the influence of androgen on FSH action switches from stimulation to inhibition as preovulatory development advances[38-40], suggesting a bimodal paracrine function for follicular androgen: stimulatory during early stages, becoming inhibitory as the follicle undergoes preovulatory development.

Androgens and Atresia

Androgens have long been associated with follicular atresia, based mainly on the inhibitory effect of androgen on oestrogen-induced granulosa cell proliferation in hypophysectomised rat ovaries[41,42]. However, such an inhibitory action of androgen has not been observed in primate ovary. On the contrary, a recent study by Vendola et al.[43] showed that follicular atresia was reduced by systemic treatment of immature rhesus monkeys with testosterone or dihydrotestosterone treatment had identical effects, indicating that these growth-promoting actions are mediated by the androgen receptor. These findings suggest that androgens are not atretogenic and actually enhance follicular growth and survival in the primate

A high follicular fluid androgen concentration is not by itself a marker of follicular atresia but the intrafollicular hormonal milieu in large (>6 mm diameter) antral follicles is dominated by androgens when they are atretic, as opposed to oestrogen when they are healthy[44]. However, in primate ovary AR gene expression is most abundant in granulosa cells of healthy growing follicles, where its expression is up-regulated by testosterone[45]. The positive correlation between granulosa AR gene expression and cell proliferation and negative correlation with programmed cell death suggests that androgens stimulate early primate follicle development.

Conclusion: a Working Hypothesis

The discovery that the granulosa cell AR system is developmentally regulated may help explain why both stimulatory (trophic) and inhibitory (atretic) effects have been ascribed to follicular androgens. Any factor that alters intracellular cAMP levels is a potential modulator of granulosa cell differentiation and hence follicular development. Androgen appears to modulate gonadotropin action on granulosa cells through amplification of cAMP-mediated post-receptor signalling[28,33]. As mentioned earlier, high concentrations of cAMP suppress granulosa cell proliferation and down-regulate low-tone cAMP-response genes in both rat[7] and human[46,47] granulosa cells. During early/intermediate stages of follicular development locally produced androgen acts via granulosa cell AR to promote FSH-induced granulosa cell proliferation and differentiation through amplifying cAMP-mediated post-receptor signalling. During late preovulatory follicular development, high concentrations of cAMP caused by the LH surge suppress granulosa cell proliferation and down-regulate some of the genes induced by FSH at earlier stages of maturity, including P450arom[48]. The high level of cAMP formation induced by LH also induces cellular changes leading to luteinisation – notably onset of progesterone syn-

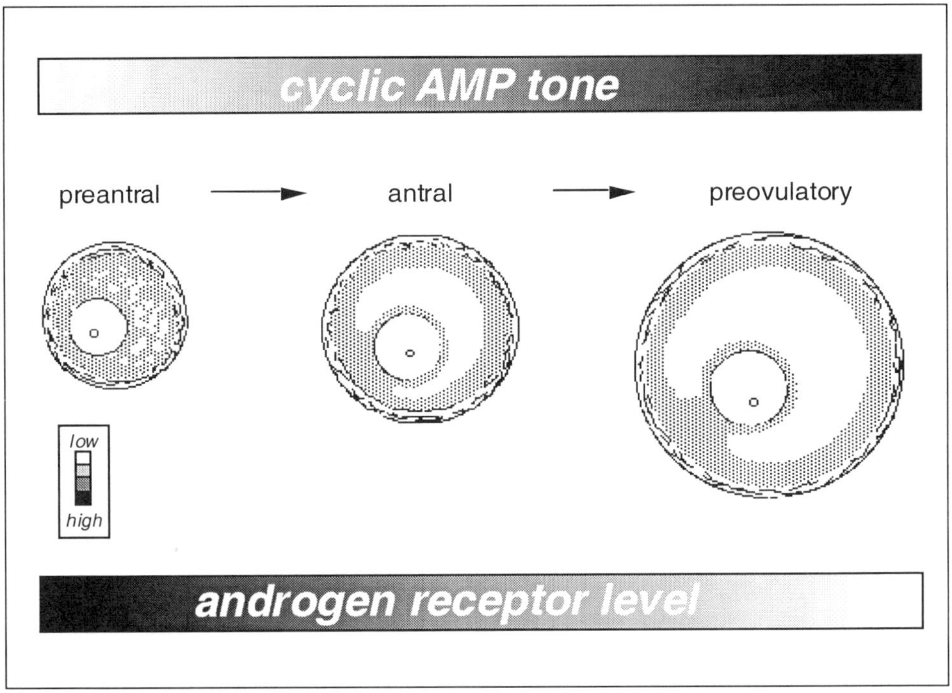

FIGURE 1 - *Schematic interaction between granulosa cell cAMP 'tone' and androgen receptor level during follicular development in the mammalian ovary, which may help explain why both stimulatory (tropic) and inhibitory (atretic) effects have been ascribed to follicular androgens. During preovulatory follicular maturation androgen receptor levels in granulosa cells decline whereas cAMP levels rise. It is proposed that during early/intermediate follicular development regulated by FSH, androgens act via granulosa cell androgen receptors to amplify cAMP-mediated granulosa cell differentiation. During late preovulatory follicular development, high concentrations of cAMP stimulated by LH suppress granulosa cell proliferation and induce luteinisation. A development related loss of androgen receptors may be part of a paracrine mechanism that reduces granulosa cell responsiveness to LH (cAMP), affording protection against premature luteinisation and atresia.* (Reproduced, with permission from Reference 3).

thesis – and terminates follicular growth through suppressing granulosa cell proliferation[45,46]. Hyperstimulation of intracellular cAMP levels before a follicle reaches full maturity may thereby initiate atresia. The experimental evidence from studies of rat and non-human primate ovaries discussed above indicates that AR levels in granulosa cells decline during preovulatory follicular maturation. Since androgens augment FSH-induced cAMP formation, loss of AR could be a means of avoiding inappropriately high cAMP levels and hence premature activation of 'high-tone' cAMP-response genes, leading to atresia (Figure 1). Thus negative regulation of the granulosa cell AR could be part of the intraovarian mechanism that determines which follicle(s) becomes dominant and secretes oestrogen in the normal menstrual cycle.

Acknowledgements

Supported by MRC Programme Grant No. 8929853

References

1. Hillier S.G.: Hormonal control of folliculogenesis and luteinisation. In: Findlay JK. (ed). *Molecular Biology of the Female Reproductive System.* Academic Press, New York, pp. 1-37, 1994.
2. Richards J.S.: Hormonal Control of gene expression in the ovary. *Endocr. Rev.*, 15:725-751, 1994.
3. Hillier S.G., Tetsuka M.: Role of androgens in follicle maturation and atresia. *Baillieres Clin. Obstet. Gynaecol.*, 11:249-260, 1997.
4. Hillier S.G.: Regulatory functions for inhibin and activin in human ovaries. *J. Endocr.*, 131:171-175, 1991.
5. Zeleznik A.J., Hillier S.G.: The ovary: endocrine function. In: Hillier S.G., Kitchener H.C., Neilson J.M. (eds), *Scientific Essentials of Reproductive Medicine.* WB Saunders, London, pp. 133-146, 1996.
6. Ross G.T.: Disorders of the ovary and female reproductive tract. In: Wilson J.D., Foster D.W. (eds), *Williams Textbook of Endocrinology*, seventh edition. WB Saunders, London, pp. 206-257, 1985.
7. Baird D.T.: Synthesis and secretion of steroid hormones by the ovary in vivo. In: Zuckerman S., Weir B.J. (eds), *The Ovary*, Vol III, second edition. Academic Press, London, pp. 305-307, 1977.
8. Dowsett M., Cantwell B., Anshumala L., Jeffcoated S.L., Harris A.: Suppression of postmenopausal ovarian steroidogenesis with the luteinizing hormone-releasing hormone agonist Gosrelin. *J. Clin. Endocrinol. Metab.*, 66: 672-677, 1988.
9. Armstrong D.T., Goff A.K., Dorrington J.H.: Regulation of follicular estrogen biosynthesis. In: Midgley A.R., Sadler W.A. (eds), *Ovarian Follicular Development and Function.* Raven Press, New York, pp. 169-182, 1979.
10. Hillier S.G., Whitelaw P.F., Smyth C.D.: Follicular oestrogen synthesis: the two-cell, two-gonadotrophin model revisited. *Mol. Cell. Endocrinol.*, 100:51-54, 1994.
11. Whitelaw P.F., Smyth C.D., Howles C.M., Hillier S.G.: Cell-specific expression of aromatase and LH receptor mRNAs in rat ovary. *J. Mol. Endocrinol.*,

9:309-313, 1992.
12. Gougeon A., Lefévre B.: Evolution of the largest healthy and atretic follicles during the human menstrual cycle. *J. Reprod. Fertil.*, 69:497-502, 1983.
13. McNatty K.P., Baird D.T., Bolton A., Chambers P., Corker C.S., McLean H.: Concentration of oestrogens and androgens in human ovarian venous plasma and follicular fluid throughout the menstrual cycle. *J. Endocrinol.*, 71:77-85, 1976.
14. Hillier S.G.: Paracrine control of follicular estrogen synthesis. *Semin. Reprod. Endocrinol.*, 9:332-340, 1991.
15. Hillier S.G., Reichert L.E. Jr., van Hall E.V.: Control of preovulatory follicular estrogen biosynthesis in the human ovary. *J. Clin. Endocrinol. Metab.*, 52:847-856, 1981.
16. Smyth C.D., Miró F., Whitelaw P.F., Howles C.M., Hillier S.G.: Ovarian thecal/interstitial androgen synthesis is enhanced by a follicle-stimulating hormone-stimulated mechanism. *Endocrinology*, 133:1532-1538, 1993.
17. Hillier S.G., Wickings E.J., Illingworth P.I., Yong E.L., Reichert L.E. Jr., Baird D.T., McNeilly A.S.: Control of immunoreactive inhibin production by human granulosa cells. *Clin. Endocrinol.*, 35:71-78, 1991.
18. Hillier S.G., Yong E.L., Illingworth P.J., Baird D.T., Schwall R.H., Mason A.J. Effect of recombinant inhibin on androgen synthesis in cultured human thecal cells. *Mol. Cell. Endocrinol.*, 75:R1-R6, 1991.
19. Adashi E.Y., Resnick C.E., Hernandez E..R, May J.V., Knecht M., Svoboda M.E., Van Wyk J.J.: Insulin-like growth factor-I as an amplifier of follicle-stimulating hormone action: studies on mechanism(s) and site(s) of action in cultured rat granulosa cells. *Endocrinology*, 122:1583-1591, 1988.
20. Van der Hoek K.H., Woodhouse C.M., Brannstrom M., Norman R.J.: Effects of interleukin (IL)-6 on luteinizing hormone- and IL-1beta-induced ovulation and steroidogenesis in the rat ovary. *Biol. Reprod.*, 58:1266-1271, 1998.
21. Roy S.K., Kole A.R.: Ovarian transforming growth factor-beta (TGF-beta) receptors: in-vitro effects of follicle stimulating hormone, epidermal growth factor and TGF-beta on receptor expression in human preantral follicles. *Mol. Hum. Reprod.*, 4:207-214, 1998.
22. Dorrington J., Chuma A.V., Bendell J.J.: Transforming growth factor-ß and follicle-stimulating hormone promote rat granulosa cell proliferation. *Endocrinology*, 123:353-359, 1988.
23. Li Ronghao, Phillips D.M., Mather J.P.: Activin promotes ovarian follicle development in vitro. *Endocrinology*, 136:849-856, 1995.
24. Miró F., Hillier S.G.: Modulation of granulosa cell deoxyribonucleic acid synthesis and differentiation by activin. *Endocrinology*, 137: 464-469, 1996.

25. Dong J., Albertini D.F., Nishimori K., Kumar T.R., Lu N., Matzuk M.M.: Growth differentiation factor-9 is required during early ovarian folliculogenesis. *Nature*, 383:531-535, 1996.
26. Parrott J.A., Skinner M.K.: Thecal cell-granulosa cell interactions involve a positive feedback loop among keratinocyte growth factor, hepatocyte growth factor, and Kit ligand during ovarian follicular development. *Endocrinology*, 139:2240-2245, 1998.
27. de Jong F.H., Grootenhuis A.J., Klaij I.A., van Beurden W.M.O.: Inhibin and related proteins: localisation, regulation and effects. In: Porter J.C., Jezova D. (eds), *Circulating Regulatory Factors and Neuroendocrine Function.* Plenum Press, New York, pp. 271-293, 1990.
28. Hillier S.G.: Intrafollicular paracrine function of ovarian androgen. *J. Steroid. Biochem.*, 27:351-357, 1987.
29. Daniel S.A.J., Armstrong D.T.: Enhancement of follicle stimulating hormone-induced aromatase activity by androgens in cultured rat granulosa cells. *Endocrinology*, 107:1027-1033, 1980.
30. Hillier S.G., de Zwart F.A.. Evidence that granulosa cell aromatase induction/activation by FSH is an androgen receptor regulated process *in vitro.* *Endocrinology*, 109:1303-1305, 1981.
31. Schreiber J.R., Reid R., Ross G.T.: A receptor-like testosterone binding protein in ovaries from estrogen-stimulated hypophysectomized immature female rats. *Endocrinology*, 98:1206-1213, 1976.
32. Schreiber J.R., Ross G.T.: Further characterisation of a rat ovarian testosterone receptor with evidence of nuclear translocation. *Endocrinology*, 99:590-596, 1997.
33. Fitzpatrick S.L., Richards J.S.: Regulation of cytochrome P450 aromatase messenger ribonucleic acid and activity by steroids and gonadotropins in rat granulosa cells. *Endocrinology*, 129:1452-1462, 1991.
34. Hillier S.G., de Zwart F.A.: Androgen/antiandrogen modulation of cyclic AMP-induced steroidogenesis during granulosa cell differentiation in tissue culture. *Mol. Cell. Endocrinol.*, 28:347-361, 1982.
35. Tetsuka M., Hillier S.G.: Androgen receptor gene expression in rat granulosa cells: the role of follicle-stimulating hormone and steroid hormones. *Endocrinology*, 137:4392-4397, 1996.
36. Tetsuka M., Whitelaw P.F., Bremner W.J., Millar M.R., Smyth C.D., Hillier S.G.: Developmental regulation of androgen receptor in rat ovary. *J. Endocrinol.*, 145:535-543, 1995.
37. Hillier S.G., Tetsuka M., Fraser H.M.: Location and developmental regulation of androgen receptor in primate ovary. *Hum. Reprod.*, 12:107-110, 1997.

38. Harlow C.R., Hillier S.G., Hodges J.K.: Androgen modulation of follicle-stimulating hormone induced granulosa cell steroidogenesis in the primate ovary. *Endocrinology*, 119:1403-1405, 1986.
39. Harlow C.R., Shaw H.G., Hillier S.G., Hodges J.K.: Factors influencing follicle-stimulating hormone-responsive steroidogenesis in marmoset granulosa cells: effects of androgens and the stage of follicular maturity. *Endocrinology*, 122:2780-2787, 1988.
40. Shaw H.G., Hillier S.G., Hodges J.K.: Developmental changes in luteinizing hormone/human chorionic gonadotropin steroidogenic responsiveness in marmoset granulosa cells: effects of follicle-stimulating hormone and androgens. *Endocrinology*, 124:1669-1677, 1989.
41. Hillier S.G., Zeleznik A.J., Knazek R.A., Ross G.T.: Hormonal regulation preovulatory follicle maturation in the rat. *J. Reprod. Fertil.*, 60:219-229, 1980.
42. Billig H., Furuta I., Hsueh A.J.W.: Estrogens inhibit and androgens enhance ovarian granulosa cell apoptosis. *Endocrinology*, 13:2204-2212, 1993.
43. Vendola K.A., Zhou J., Adesanya O.O., Weil S.J., Bondy C.A.: Androgens stimulate early stages of follicular growth in the primate ovary. *Clin. Invest.*, 101:2622-2629, 1998.
44. Westergaard L., Christensen I.J., McNatty K.P.: Steroid levels in ovarian follicular fluid related to follicle size and health status during the normal menstrual cycle in women. *Human Reproduction*, 1:227-232, 1986.
45. Weil S.J., Vendola K., Zhou J., Adesanya O.O., Wang J., Okafor J., Bondy C.A.: Androgen receptor gene expression in the primate ovary: cellular localization, regulation, and functional correlations. *J. Clin. Endocrinol. Metab.*, 83:2479-2485,1998.
46. Yong E.L., Baird D.T., Hillier S.G.: Mediation of gonadotrophin-stimulated growth and differentiation of human granulosa cells by adenosine 3',5'-monophosphate: one molecule, two messages. *Clin. Endocrinol.*, 37:51-58, 1992.
47. Yong E.L., Baird D.T., Yates R., Reichert L.E. Jr., Hillier S.G.: Hormonal regulation of the growth and steroidogenic function of human granulosa cells. *J. Clin. Endocrinol. Metab.*, 74:842-849, 1992.
48. Yong E.L., Hillier S.G., Turner M., Baird D.T., Ng S.C., Bongso A., Ratnam S.S.: Differential regulation of cholesterol side-chain cleavage (P450scc) and aromatase (P450arom) enzyme mRNA expression by gonadotrophins and cyclic AMP in human granulosa cells. *J. Mol. Endocrinol.*, 12:239-249, 1994.

The Role of Luteinizing Hormone
in Folliculogenesis
and Ovulation Induction, pp. 79-89
Editor M. Filicori

Serum Hormone Dynamics Following Different Menotropin Regimens

R. Fleming

*University Department of Obstetrics and Gynaecology
Royal Infirmary, Glasgow (United Kingdom)*

Abstract. *Ovarian responses to exogenous stimulation are influenced by a number of components; including the circulating LH concentrations, drug (FSH) potency and kinetics. Purified urinary FSH can be administered sub-cutaneously, which yields different circulating concentration profiles, which may influence ovarian responses, and also dose requirements.*

Complete LH suppression is not achieved during GnRH-A treatment for controlled ovarian hyperstimulation (COH), and in most cases there is sufficient circulating LH to allow E_2 biosynthesis to proceed in response to FSH alone. However, purified FSH yields less E_2 in the circulation than does HMG, and cases where the endogenous LH is suppressed to a more profound degree show less E_2 in the circulation and lower concentrations of testosterone (T) and E_2 in the follicular fluid. In these cycles, the circulating inhibin-B concentration is unaffected, showing that the number of small follicles recruited is similar, but the inhibin-A values are reduced in the late follicular phase of cycles with more profoundly suppressed LH suggesting that the degree of development of larger follicles may be reduced where the LH activity is low.

In COH for IVF, the circulating progesterone (P) concentrations may be seen to rise prior to HCG administration without indications of increased LH activity. This has been termed "premature luteinization" although there is no indication of luteinization of ovarian tissue. It occurs in cycles treated with either HMG or FSH. Furthermore, in cycles treated with FSH, when LH was added in the late follicular phase, a significant increase in E_2, but no change in P secretion was observed. This indicates that the phenomenon is unrelated to normal luteinization processes.

Key words. Follicle growth, FSH, inhibin, premature luteinisation.

Introduction

The demand for exogenous stimulation with follicle stimulating hormone (FSH) has paralleled the rapid rise of the treatment of infertility with IVF and its related processes. In the 1980's, human menopausal gonadotropins (hMG), containing both FSH and luteinizing hormone (LH) was the universal stimulant used in controlled ovarian stimulation (COS) programmes where LH surges were eliminated using GnRH-analogs (GnRH-a). The combined therapy was responsible for the high yield of oocytes upon which the success of IVF depends so strongly.

Recent technological advances allowed the introduction of purified menotropins which enjoy much reduced contamination from numerous urinary protein products and also much greater specific activity[1]. This, in turn, allows subcutaneous (s.c.) administration, effectively reducing clinical stress as patients often self-administer and are required to attend the clinic less frequently. The purification processing of the urinary extract may reduce the batch-to-batch variation seen in the more traditional hMG and FSH preparations, but it does not do so to the standards seen in the newer, more expensive, recombinant preparations (rFSH).

The changes in the menotropin preparations can impact on the physiology at 3 levels. Firstly, the pharmacokinetics of circulating FSH concentrations appears to depend on the site (mode) of administration. Secondly, the iso-

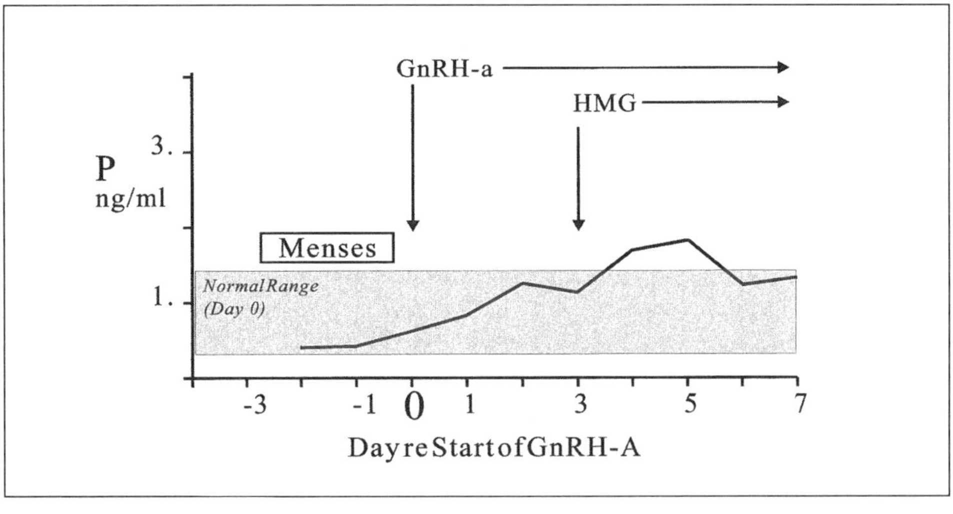

FIGURE 1 - *Progesterone (P) in the first week of treatment in patients treated with hMG, in a short course programme.*

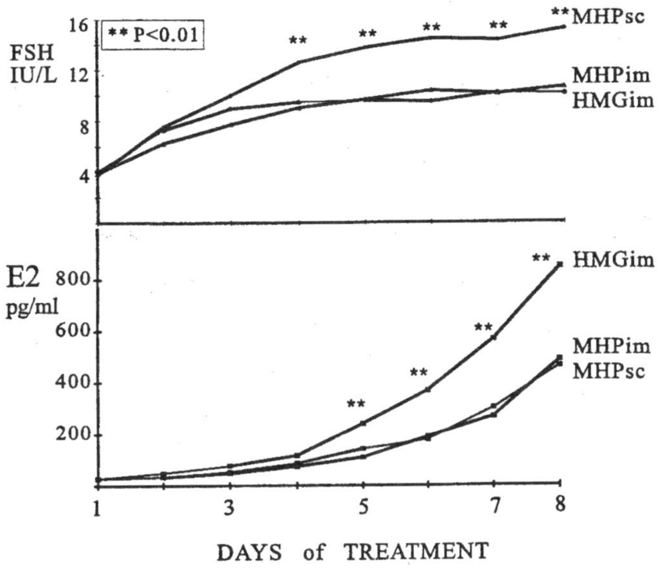

FIGURE 2 - *Mean FSH and E2 profiles in the first week of treatment in patients treated with purified FSH (MHP) or hMG.*

form profile of the FSH preparation influences both end-target tissue responses and clearance rates, which of course influence the pharmacokinetics. Thirdly, the elimination of LH from the stimulation preparation influences ovarian responses in women with no or suppressed endogenous gonadotrophin output, depending on the circumstances (see chapter 15).

Variations in hormone profiles also depend upon the particular stimulation regimen used, as the absence of LH in the stimulant will be less important with the short course GnRH-a administration, which utilises the flare effect at the start of treatment. Here, the LH is rarely fully suppressed by the time of HCG administration, and is therefore unlikely to influence follicular development during the follicular phase. However, in these cycles the endogenous gonadotrophin surge in the flare response can become critical, as it can rescue the corpus luteum, or luteinize any early developing follicles, depending when the treatment is started in reference to the ovarian cycle. Figure 1 shows the mean responses of progesterone (P) to the flare effect in a short course programme with the analog starting on cycle day 3. Some of the individuals within the group showed P concentrations above the cycle normal value for more than 3 days. We may expect that this would have implications at the level of the endometrium, if not at the ovary or oocyte. Profiles such as these may explain the apparent reduced success of short coarse cycles. For this reason, and the fact that the majority of assisted reproduction cycles are effected using the long coarse GnRH-a protocols, the remainder of this paper will concentrate on the standard long coarse protocol which has been used widely since 1982[2].

FSH Pharmacokinetics

There is little difference in the pharmacokinetic properties of the FSH from preparations of similar origin, such that the highly purified FSH (Metrodin-HP, Laboratoires Serono, Switzerland) showed profiles of absorption and clearance that were indistinguishable from those of simple urinary FSH (Metrodin, Laboratoires Serono). However, although the total bio-availability of s.c. and intramuscular administration were similar (close to 100%) the Tmax was delayed in the s.c. group after bolus administration[3,4], and the distribution curve appeared to be shifted to the right. Repeated daily administration, therefore, may lead to different concentration profiles more related to the mode and site of administrations than to the specific preparation. Figure 2 shows that repeated daily injections of purified FSH administered s.c., achieves higher circulating immunoassayable FSH concentrations than the

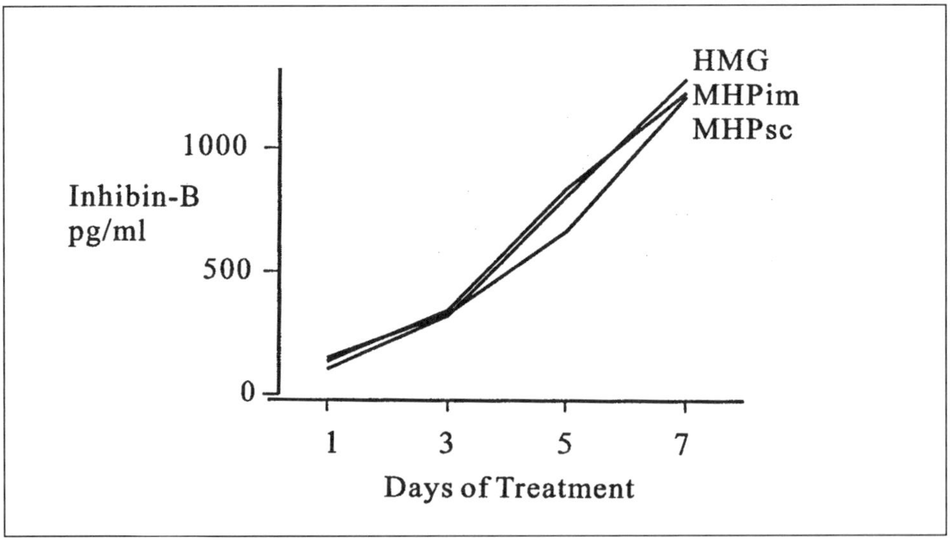

FIGURE 3 - *Circulating mean concentrations of inhibin-B in the first week of treatment in patients treated with purified FSH (MHP) or hMG.*

i.m. injection, and these peak concentrations are achieved by day 4 of treatment irrespective of the product or the route of administration[5].

During the regimen of once daily administration, there are peak and trough concentrations, but the dynamics of follicular responses to this type of hormone concentration profile are not well understood. However, there appears to be a threshold value of FSH sensitivity for each individual follicle, and it is not clear whether the number of follicles recruited is more related to peak, mean, or trough values experienced within the 24h cycle. However, there is a well established pattern that higher doses of FSH yield more follicles, within certain limits. Figure 2 shows that the s.c. administration of purified FSH (MHPsc) yielded higher concentration profiles than the i.m., but there was no difference seen in follicular recruitment patterns as demonstrated by the E2 profiles. Figure 3 shows the profiles of inhibin-B in the same groups of patients treated with HMG or FSH, related to the mode of administration. Inhibin-B is generally thought to be a product of the small recruited follicle, and the concentration profiles showed no difference with respect to the site of administration, or the FSH preparation. The degree of small follicle recruitment, represented by inhibin-B, was identical in all groups. Thus, the lower E_2 concentrations seen in both the MHP groups compared with the HMG group (Figure 2) probably reflect the difference in the degree of LH stimulation, not the drug pharmacokinetics or dynamics.

In the study shown in Figures 2 and 3, a daily dose of 225 IU/day FSH was administered, but despite the differences seen in the circulating FSH concentrations, there was no difference in the number of follicles recruited, the duration of treatment, or the number of oocytes retrieved. Thus, this dose probably represented excess stimulation in the majority of cases, as recruitment was generally at its maximum. Analyses of the circulating inhibin-A concentrations in these cycles at the time of HCG administration (mean values: HMGim = 1100; MHPim = 1150; MHPsc = 1540 ng/ml) also showed no differences between the treatment groups. Thus, the numbers of larger follicles recruited in the FSH treated cycles appears to be unrelated to the source and administration of FSH, when given at these doses.

However, the E_2 profiles did show differences related to the circulating follicular phase LH, and this may have a more profound effect upon follicular recruitment and development than anything else (see chapter 15).

FSH Isoforms

Native FSH is a glycoprotein hormone constituted from two polypeptide subunits, both of which are linked to carbohydrate chains which vary considerably and which confer a spectrum of biochemical and biological properties upon the molecules. The structures of the carbohydrate chains confer all the qualitative variations in the molecule, and target cell function is strongly influenced by the receptor binding capacities of the particular iso-hormones present.

Fractions of FSH isoforms are released from chromatographic columns according to their molecular charges, and different iso-hormone profiles are observed for urinary and recombinant products. All fractions are acidic, due to the sialic acid components of the carbohydrate chains, and they are released from the column at pH values from around 6 down to 2.5[6].

The higher the pI of the FSH fraction (i.e. less acidic), the higher its Bioactivity / Immuno-activity ratio and its target cell binding affinity. These fractions, or isoforms, show a considerably greater ability to elicit responses in a variety of target cell bio-assays. So the greatest in-vitro activity is seen in the least acidic fractions. However, these fractions are also cleared from the circulation more rapidly than the acidic ones, so the in vivo activity of a particular preparation may depend more on the content of the more acidic components. Urinary FSH products show greater batch-to-batch variation in the

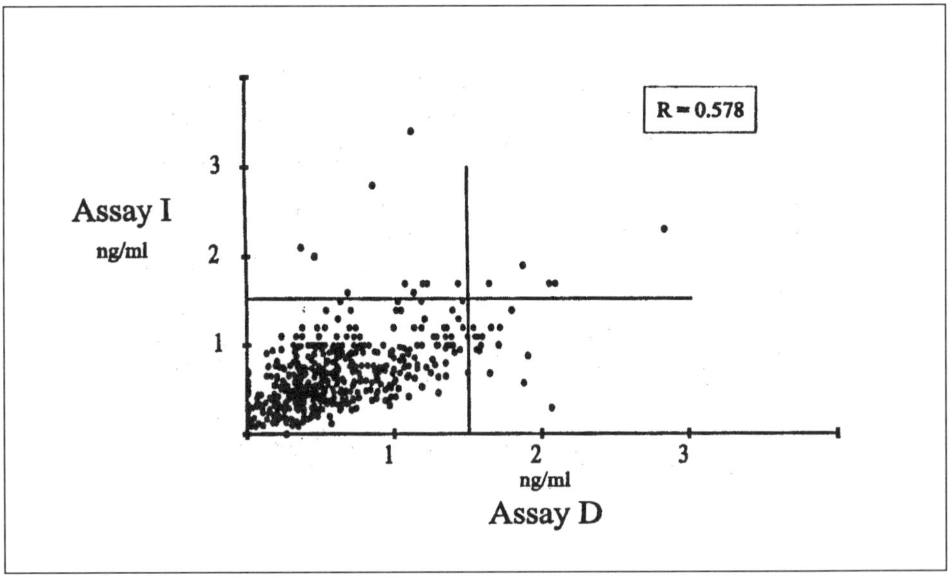

FIGURE 4 - *Scatter plot of the concentrations of P in late follicular phase plasma samples effected using 2 different commercial assays. Determination of values >1.5 ng/ml showed a poor correlation.*

isoform profiles than the recombinant products, and they show a higher proportion of the more acidic products. Although, these factors are difficult to study in the clinical setting, it is probable that the higher proportion of the basic isoforms found in recombinant FSH is responsible for its apparent higher potency.

Follicular Phase Progesterone Secretion

During COS cycles, pituitary desensitisation with GnRH-a eliminates both immunoactive and bioactive LH surges, but the circulating progesterone (P) concentrations may be seen to undergo a subtle rise prior to HCG administration, and some authors associate this phenomenon with adverse treatment outcome. Reduced implantation and pregnancy rates have been reported, although these are controversial observations. The rise in P has been termed "premature luteinization"[7], which suggests that it originates from differentiation mechanisms of cells in the stimulated follicles: as if in response to a luteinizing signal. It has been suggested that it may be caused by the LH component or small amounts of contaminant HCG in the menotropin preparation.

Technical Observations. One of the problems with these investigations is the limitation of the assays used to investigate the changes of P concentrations at the low concentration ranges seen in the follicular phase. Figure 4 shows that there is little agreement between two of the commercial assays in these follicular phase samples, and this concept may account for some of the disagreements between publications on this issue. Furthermore, because the different assays are clearly detecting different environments in different patients, it is difficult to confirm that the phenomenon is of real biological significance or merely technical artefact. Recovery examinations of the different assays at these low concentrations do not provide the confidence required to examine the phenomenon with great exactitude. However, within patient control can be used for etiological studies, if not for determination of valid physiological phenomena in large populations.

The Role of LH in Follicular Phase P Elevations. In order to determine if the LH (or HCG) component of hMG was responsible for the increased P seen in the circulation prior to HCG administration, we examined the effects of additional LH, in the form of hMG, as a substitute for purified FSH in the final 2 days of stimulation. The patients were monitored with ultrasound examinations and when the leading follicle was > 14mm the patient was rand-

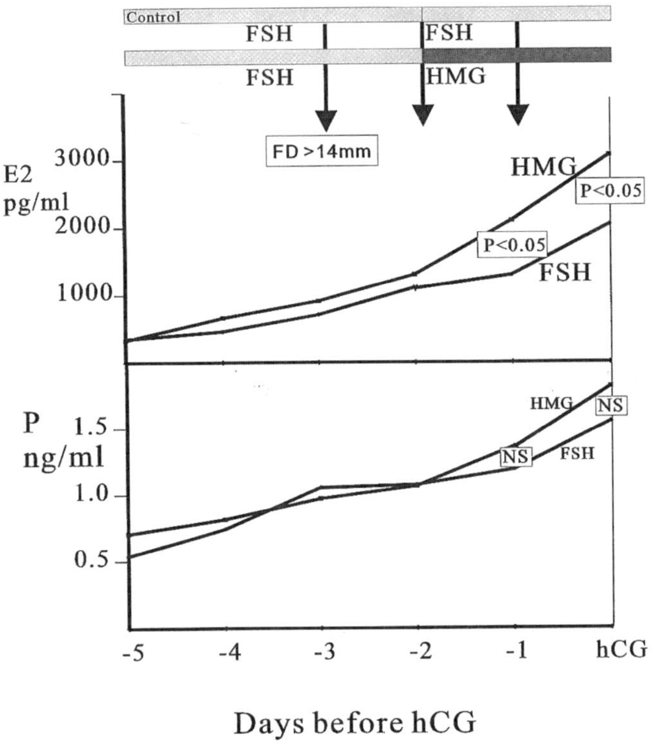

FIGURE 5 - *Changes in E_2 and P at the end of the follicular phase of COS cycles stimulated initially with purified FSH, and finally without or with (hMG) a component of LH.*

omized to receive either hMG or purified FSH for the final 2 days prior to HCG. The exposure to FSH was similar in both groups.

Figure 5 shows that after the change to hMG there was a significant increase in E2 relative to the control group receiving FSH all through the follicular phase. Both groups showed a continued rise in E_2, but the hMG treated women showed an immediate and significantly greater increase after the change in stimulant[8]. This observation reflects the 2-cell/2-gonadotrophin mechanism of E_2 biosynthesis in the follicles at this time. However, figure 5 also shows no increase in the P concentrations in the peripheral circulation of the women treated with hMG compared with the controls receiving FSH alone.

It has been suggested that the subtle rise in P in the late follicular phase may be related to the use of the nasal spray mode of administration of the GnRH-A, allowing sufficient LH fluctuations to cause luteinization[9]. It was also suggested[10] that the etiology of the subtle rise in P may be related to an increased LH sensitivity of the granulosa cells of FSH treated cycles.

This simple experiment shows that the inclusion of a luteinising component into the stimulation of GnRH-A cycles over the final 2 days failed to influence the circulating P concentrations. This indicates that the "premature luteinization" or increases in circulating P described in cycles treated with GnRH-A are unrelated to any normally recognised luteinising process, including LH-sensitized follicular cells. It is more likely that the increases are caused by increased total output of P by two highly stimulated, but unluteinised ovaries.

If the hypotheses describing a luteinizing process were the correct explanation of the late follicular phase increase in P concentrations, then the introduction of a late follicular phase LH component would have caused an increase in the circulating concentration of P: not so.

With regard to the hypothesis that the subtle rise in progesterone may be due to lack of catabolism of progesterone through to E_2, the data do not support this hypothesis either. The significant increase in E_2, with no change in the P suggests that the etiology of the observation is neither based upon luteinization nor altered follicular catabolism of P.

The ovarian vein draining the ovary with the dominant follicle, shows P concentrations that are considerably higher than the peripheral circulation through most of the follicular phase of the normal cycle. It would be expected that 2 highly stimulated ovaries, as seen in IVF cycles, would carry large quantities into the circulation. The normal clearance rates at this level may also show individual variations between subjects, and minor increases in P may be due to a combination of increased non-luteinised ovarian output and limited clearance rate.

The rapid and significant response of the circulating E_2 to the introduction of the LH component is further evidence that the E_2 secretion by the ovaries in GnRH-A cycles treated with purified FSH is sub-normal. The data support other observations that purified FSH fails to induce the expected output of E_2 in IVF cycles in normal women treated with a GnRH-analog. The reasons for the sub-optimal E_2 secretion are probably related to insufficient androgen biosynthesis by the follicular theca cells in response to LH as seen in women with hypogonadotrophic hypogonadism[12]. The speed of the response suggests that the aromatase enzyme system was established and merely starved of the androgen precursor.

The conclusion that this phenomenon is not due to any form of luteinization implies that there can be no basis for any influence upon oocyte or embryo developmental competence. This would support the conclusion of a comprehensive clinical study indicating that there was no effect of "premature luteinization" upon implantation and pregnancy rates in IVF[13].

These data indicate that, if the phenomenon has real biological implications, then its aetiology should be sought in areas unrelated to the luteinizing components of the menotropins.

Conclusions

After all this time of routine exogenous gonadotrophin therapy with GnRH-a co-treatment, the endocrinology and pharmacology remain important factors in the success of IVF. The newer gonadotrophin preparations do present new challenges, and our approaches to monitoring responses have to be modified. Purified urinary FSH allows self-administration, yielding higher concentrations, and maybe lower doses to attain similar degrees of follicular growth. On the other hand, the isoform profile suggests that the acidic bias of this product would imply lower tissue stimulation activity. However, its use does suffer from the same uncontrolled variable as recombinant FSH administration in COS-low endogenous LH activity. This impacts upon circulating E_2 concentrations and follicular fluid testosterone and E_2 levels. The subtle rise in P seen at the end of the follicular phase, however, appears to be unrelated to the LH activity.

References

1. Giudice E., Crisci C., Eshkol A., Papoian R.: Composition of commercial gonadotrophin preparations extracted from human post-menopausal urine: characterization of non-gonadotrophin proteins. *Hum. Reprod.*, 9:2291-2299, 1994.
2. Fleming R., Adams A.H., Barlow D.H., Black W.P., Macnaughton M.C., Coutts J.R.T.: A new systematic treatment for infertile women with abnormal hormone profiles. *Brit. J. Obstet. Gynaecol.*, 80:80-83. 1982.
3. Le Cotonnec J.-Y., Porchet H.C., Beltrami V., Howles C.: Comparative pharmacokinetics of two urinary follicle stimulating hormone preparations in healthy female and male volunteers. *Hum. Reprod.*, 8:1604-1611, 1993.
4. Dobbs K.E., Dumesic D.A., Dumesic J.A., Shapiro S.S.: Differences in serum follicle stimulating hormone uptake after intramuscular and subcutaneous human menoipausal gonadotropin injection. *Fertil. Steril.*, 62:978-983, 1994.

5. Fleming R., Chung C.C., Yates R.W.S., Coutts J.R.T.: Purified urinary follicle stimulating hormone induces different hormone profiles compared with menotrophins, dependent upon route of administration and endogenous luteinizing hormone activity. *Hum. Reprod.*, 11:1854-1858, 1996.
6. De Leeuw R., Mulders J., Voortman G., Rombout F., Damm J., Klosterboer L.: Structure-function relationship of recombinant follicle stimulating hormone (Puregon). *Hum. Reprod.*, 2:361-369, 1996.
7. Silverberg K.M., Burns W.N., Olive D.L., Riehl R.M., Shenken R.S.: Serum progesterone levels predict success of in vitro fertilisation/embryo transfer in patients stimulated with leuprolide acetate and human menopausal gonadotropins. *J. Clin. Endocr. and Metab.*, 73:797-803, 1991.
8. Adonakis G., Deshpande N., Yates R.W.S., Fleming R.: Luteinizing hormone increases estradiol secretion but has no effect on progesterone concentrations in the late follicular phase of in vitro fertilization cycles in women treated with gonadotropin releasing hormone agonis. *Fertil. Steril.*, 69:450-453, 1998.
9. Filicori M.: Letter-to-the-editor. *Fertil. Steril.*, 67:1179, 1997.
10. McNatty K.P., Baird D.T., Bolton A., Chambers P., Corker C.S., Mclean H.: Concentration of oestrogens and androgens in human ovarian venous plasma and follicular fluid throughout the menstrual cycle. *J. Endocrinol.*, 71:77, 1976.
11. Ubaldi F., Camus M., Smitz J., Coelingh Bennink H., van Sterteghem A., Devroey P.: Premature luteinization in in vitro fertilisation cycles using gonadotrophin releasing hormone agonist (GnRH-a) and recombinant follicle stimulating hormone (FSH) and GnRH-a and urinary FSH. *Fertil. Steril.*, 66:275-280, 1996.
12. Couzinet B., Lestrat N., Brailly S., Forest M., Schaison G.: Stimulation of ovarian follicular maturation with pure follicle stimulating hormone in women with gonadotropin deficiency. *J. Clin. Endocrinol. Metab.*, 66:552-556, 1988.
13. Hofmann G.E., Khoury J., Johnson C.A., Thie J., Scott R.T.: Premature luteinization during controlled ovarian hyperstimulation for in vitro fertilization-embryo transfer has no impact on pregnancy outcome. *Fertil. Steril.*, 66:980-986, 1996.

The Role of Luteinizing Hormone
in Folliculogenesis
and Ovulation Induction, pp. 91-104
Editor M. Filicori

Endogenous LH Secretion in Hypogonadotropic Hypogonadism

R. Quinton and H.S. Jacobs

Division of Endocrinology, UCL Medical School
Cobbold Laboratories, The Middlesex Hospital, London (United Kingdom)

Abstract. *Hypogonadotropic hypogonadism (HH) is a heterogenous condition of diverse aetiology. It may result from genetic mutations as in Kallmann's syndrome (KS), or from acquired disorders that are functional (eg weight loss) or organic (infiltrating or expanding lesions in the hypothalamic-pituitary area). In both anosmic (KS) and normosmic forms of idiopathic HH, endogenous LH secretion varies between patients and may also vary over time in the same patient. Although most patients with idiopathic HH are completely apulsatile with respect to gonadotropin release, some individuals do exhibit low-level endogenous LH secretion, which is clinically reflected in larger gonadal volumes. A syndrome of acquired idiopathic HH has recently been described in a series of adult men and we have observed one female presenting with secondary hypothalamic amenorrhoea, in whom neither body weight nor psychological well-being appeared compromised. Conversely, we have identified five males, presumed to have KS because of anosmia and severe pubertal delay and thus treated with testosterone, in whom secretion of LH and FSH subsequently recovered so that they all underwent spontaneous testicular enlargement with onset of spermatogenesis between 20-35 years of age. Whether such a sequence occurs in women with KS is unknown but probable. In clinical practice, weight/stress-related HH is essentially a female phenomenon causing amenorrhoea. Nevertheless, a similar endocrine picture does occur in men under experimental conditions of food or sleep deprivation. In patients with weight loss, there is preferential suppression of the secretion of LH compared with FSH. Low endogenous LH levels contribute both to the clinical expression of the disorder and to the response to treatment. Subnormal LH stimulation of the ovary results not only in subnormal oestrogen secretion, but also in subnormal thecal androgen secretion and hence a dearth of substrate for aromatisation. Oestrogen deficiency in these women is therefore particularly severe because of lack of follicular oestrogen secretion, lack of androgenic substrate and lack of fat tissue aromatase, together with a peturbation of oestrogen catabolism that favours production of anti-oestrogens. Ovulation-induction in women with HH is* *usually performed using pulsatile GnRH, unless there is evidence of pituitary disease. Men with HH require treatment for many months to induce spermatogenesis and therefore usually elect to be treated with gonadotropin injections. Treatment outcome is affected by the rate of endogenous LH secretion; HH males with larger initial testicular volumes, indicating greater endogenous gonadotropin production, have a better and more rapid response to treatment with respect to parameters of sperm density and quality. With the increasing use of the new generation of monohormonal "pure" FSH preparations, the amount of endogenous LH secretion in HH may need to be given greater prominence when designing of protocols for ovulation-induction.*

Key words. Hypogonadotropic hypogonadism, Kallmann's syndrome, hypothalamic amenorrhoea, leptin, GnRH.

Introduction

Hypogonadotropic hypogonadism (HH) is a heterogeneous condition of diverse aetiology. It may result from genetic mutations or acquired disorders that are functional (eg weight loss) or organic (eg infiltrating or expanding lesions in the hypothalamic-pituitary area) (Table 1). In this review, while discussing several of the responsible conditions, we focus particular attention on the problems presented by patients with Kallmann's syndrome (KS) and those with weight related amenorrhoea. We have so decided because of the several advances that have been made recently in our understanding of these two conditions, their management and the light they shed on gonadotropin secretion.

HH is diagnosed by the coexistence of low serum concentrations of sex steroids and of pituitary gonadotropins. The term isolated or idiopathic hypogonadotrophic hypogonadism (IHH) implies, first, the absence of any structural lesion of the hypothalamo-pituitary unit and, second, that secretion of the other hypophyseal hormones is unaffected. In virtually all cases, IHH results from a congenital deficiency of gonadotrophin-releasing hormone (GnRH) secretion[1,2]. Exceptions include adrenohypoplasia congenita, where there is a combined defect of hypothalamic GnRH and of pituitary gonadotropin secretion[3], and those patients who harbour GnRH receptor gene mutations[4,5].

Acquired HH usually comes to medical attention earlier in women than men, because it is associated with a definite clinical event: cessation of menstruation. Conversely, in congenital HH, the external signs of delayed puberty may be less obvious in girls than boys. Furthermore, girls with primary amenorrhoea may receive empirical therapy with the oral contraceptive pill from physicians or gynaecologists in the primary care setting. An intriguing point

TABLE 1 - *Causes of hypogonadotropic hypogonadism.*

Syndrome	*Gene*
Congenital	
Hpg mouse -no human homologue[9]	*GnRH-1*
Kallmann's syndrome (anosmia)	*KAL* in X-KS[10,11] autosomal loci unknown
normosmic IHH	unknown 98% *GnRH-R* 2%[5]
adrenohypoplasia congenita	*DAX-1*[12,13]
leptin deficiency (mouse and human obesity)	*OB*[14]
leptin resistance (mouse and human obesity)	*Leptin-R*[15]
prohormone convertase-1 deficiency (obesity & hypocortisolaemia in mouse and human)	*PC-1*[16]
Gordon Holmes (spinocerebellar ataxia)[17,18]	autosomal dominant
septo-optic dysplasia (mouse and human)	*HESX-1*[19]
Acquired	
leptin deficiency (underweight)	
hypothalamo-pituitary damage (tumour, granuloma, infarction, surgery, irradiation)	
stress / systemic illness	
hyperprolactinaemia	
haemochromatosis[20]	
hypermelatoninaemia[21,22]	

of divergence between normal males and females is that marked gonadotropin pulsatility, similar to that of mid-puberty, is observed specifically in male neonates[6,7]. The biological function of this transient activation of the GnRH pulse generator is not known.

Figure 1 demonstrates paired plasma LH and testosterone concentrations in 124 males with congenital IHH. It suggests that a spectrum of gonadotropin deficiency exists in these patients. IHH is generally associated with complete LH and FSH apulsatility, and patients classically report absent pubertal development unless treated with exogenous androgens, gonadotrophins or GnRH. However, a proportion of patients do generate LH and FSH pulses, but these are either of abnormally low amplitude or occur solely in a nocturnal, sleep-entrained secretory pattern. In these patients group, the history is often of

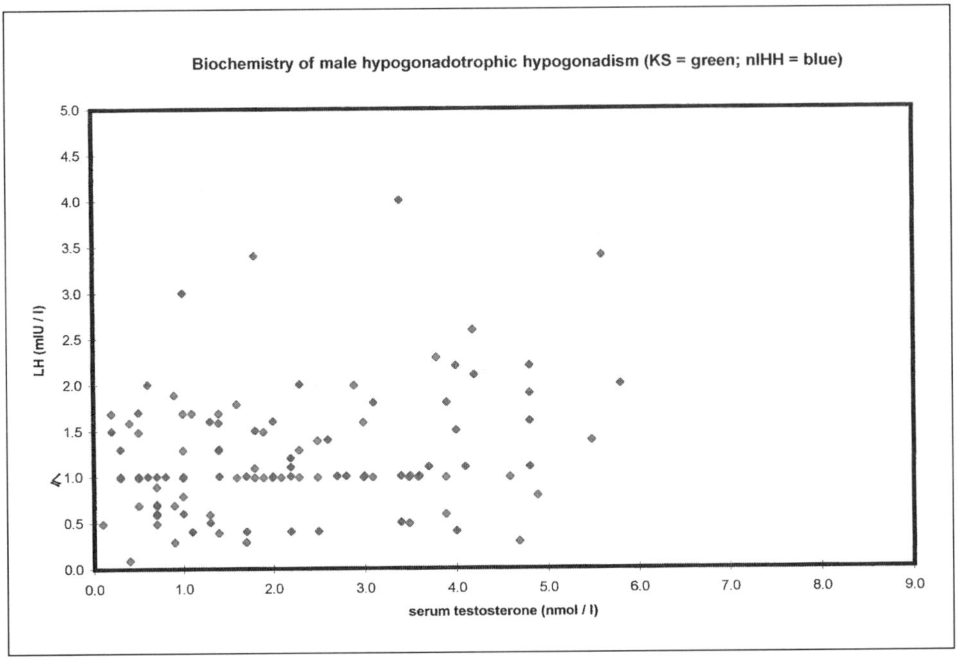

FIGURE 1 - *Scatter chart of paired plasma LH vs testosterone concentrations in IHH males.*

normal entry into puberty but with subsequent arrested development[8]. In our experience it is rarely necessary to perform 24hr LH pulsatility studies in the routine diagnosis of IHH. Gonadal volume provides an excellent assessment of integrated gonadotropin secretion and is readily assessed manually in men and ultrasonographically in women.

Kallmann's Syndrome and Isolated Hypogonadotropic Hypogonadism

GnRH-immunoreactive neurones originate outside the CNS in the developing olfactory placode and migrate intracranially along fascicles of the 1st cranial nerve complex[23]. Examination of a single 19 week male fetus, with a large terminal deletion of the X chromosomal spanning the *KAL* locus, revealed failure of these axon fascicles to penetrate the forebrain meninges, with consequent extracranial migration-arrest of GnRH neurons[24]. This finding underpins the anosmia and GnRH-deficiency of X-linked KS, but cannot be extrapolated to explain the pathophysiology of autosomal KS, nor of normosmic

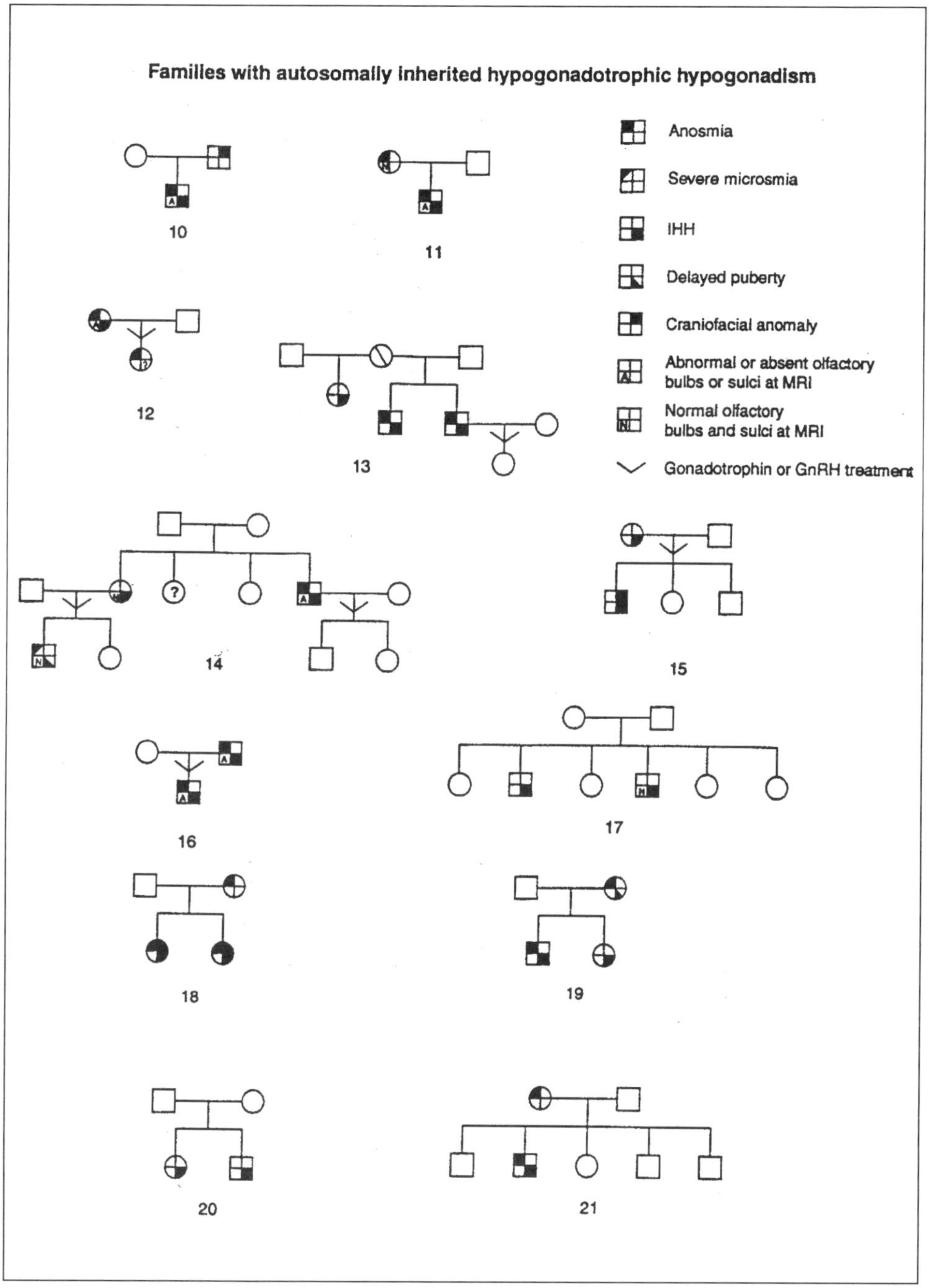

FIGURE 2 - *Autosomal IHH pedigrees.*

IHH. Table 1 illustrates how the genetic basis for most cases of IHH remains unknown. Despite the excess of affected males, which might suggest a preponderance of X-linked KS, it is estimated that no only 7-11% of sporadic KS males harbour KAL mutations or deletions[25,26].

Data on the population prevalence of IHH derive from two sources. The first was an epidemiological study of 40,000 male conscripts, all in their 20th year of age in 1971, at induction to the French army[27]. Those who appeared clinically hypogonadal on examination were investigated further by assessment of their karyotype, urinary gonadotropins and olfaction. Ten IHH cases were identified, giving a population prevalence of 0.025% and four of them had KS, hence the oft-quoted 1 in 10,000 prevalence of KS in the male population. The second was a retrospective literature search of published KS cases up to April 1975, in which 145 male and 27 female cases were identified, yielding an inexplicable 5:1 male/female preponderance[28].

We have studied a total of 216 patients with congenital IHH, of which 21% were female. 55% of the male cases and 38% of the females were anosmic, ie had Kallmann's Syndrome. Although most cases were sporadic, familial transmission was evident in 24%. 10 X-linked-KS and 13 autosomal pedigrees (Figure 2) were identified. Three patients with sporadic KS had received treatment to induce ovulation or spermatogenesis, resulting in IHH being inherited by their offspring. Figure 2 illustrates the phenotypic heterogeneity within families showing autosomal inheritance, with related individuals exhibiting KS, normosmic IHH and even isolated anosmia. There is likely to be a common autosomal gene, with variable phenotypic expression, underlying these three conditions. By contrast, X-linked KS is a much more homogeneous condition, with 85% of patients exhibiting mirror movements (involuntary, non-suppressible, homologous movements of one hand when the other is moved voluntarily) and 33% having unilateral renal agenesis[26].

Crowley's group recently published a series of 11 male cases who had all developed normally during childhood and puberty, but who had acquired idiopathic IHH in adult life[29]. This is not a phenomenon which we ourselves have observed, apart from one possible female case, presenting aged 20 years with secondary amenorrhoea. Although full pubertal development had occurred following menarche at the age of 13.5 years, current endometrial thickness was only 3mm by ultrasonography; cranial MRI and anterior pituitary function were all normal apart from LH 1.7 mIU/l, FSH 5.3 mIU/l, E_2 <40 pmol/l. While such an endocrine pattern would have been consistent with weight-related amenorrhoea, her BMI was in fact 29 kg/m^2.

By contrast, we have recently identified five males, originally presumed to have KS because of anosmia and severe pubertal delay, who, subsequently recovered endogenous gonadotropin secretion sufficient to normalise plasma testosterone concentrations, testicular volume and sperm density. This recovery of endocrine function was associated with three impregnations, despite their having been no treatment with gonadotrophins or GARH[30]. Whether such a phenomenon occurs in females is not known but the following case report suggests that gonadotropin secretion in IHH may vary over the course of a lifetime. Pedigree 19 in Figure 2 illustrates a brother and sister with KS and normosmic IHH respectively. Their mother is congenitally anosmic and was given estrogen replacement therapy in her early 20s for severe pubertal delay. For most of her life she was either amenorrhoeic or severely oligomenorrhoeic, apart from a phase of 2-3 years in her third decade when she twice became pregnant without any treatment. Currently aged 68 years, her plasma concentrations of LH and FSH were recently measured at 5.8 and 7.5 mIU/l respectively -well below the normal postmenopausal range.

Weight-related Amenorrhoeia

Amenorrhoea related to weight loss occurs commonly in university based gynaecological endocrine practice. The condition is important to identify because it may be associated with profound oestrogen deficiency (we have, for example, seen several patients in whom the presentation was with osteoporotic fractures). In addition there is evidence that, so far as treatment of the associated fertility is concerned, babies born to underweight women have an increased risk themselves of being underweight and also of being immature and premature[31]; more recent work indicates such children may have adverse patterns of health in later life[32]. For these reasons we have, for some years, advised that induction of ovulation in underweight women be deferred until nutrition has returned to normal. The return of fertility is usually then very prompt and medical treatment usually becomes unnecessary. Although most studies of stress or weight-related HH have been in females, there are also data on males. For instance, during five days of intense simulated combat stress and relative sleep deprivation, plasma testosterone levels in soldiers rapidly fell to a mean of 1.1 nmol/l[33].

Recent advances in our understanding of the control of body weight have helped elucidate the endocrine pathophysiology of this condition. Clinically perhaps the most relevant has been the unravelling of the role that leptin plays in the link between nutrition and reproduction[34]. Leptin, which is a helical cytokine of the tumour necrosis factor group, was originally identified as the product of the *Ob* gene in mice. This gene, isolated by positional cloning, encodes a 167 amino acid protein which interacts with a single transmembrane-domain receptor of the cytokine receptor family.

Leptin enters the central nervous system via the choroid plexus, interacts with its receptor in the hypothalamus and inhibits synthesis and release of neuropeptide Y (NPY)[35]. NPY is the most abundant neuropeptide in brain. It has various functions and is involved in regulation of circadian rhythm, the response to anxiety and stress, peripheral vascular resistance and cardiac contractility. It is the only peptide known to induce obesity through prolonged central administration. The link between leptin and the GnRH neurone is mediated through NPY[36], although some redundancy in the hypothalamic signalling pathway must be accepted because the NPY knockout mouse not only maintains normal body weight but is also fertile[37]. NPY is thought to be an important mediator of the body's response to starvation, while additional factors (melanocyte stimulating hormone and the melanocortin-4 receptor) are involved in the hypothalamic response to obesity[38]. NPY, which inhibits GnRH activity, is itself inhibited by leptin. Low levels of leptin are therefore associated with reduced GnRH stimulated gonadotropin secretion.

The leptin deficient (*ob/ob*) mouse is infertile, with subnormal gonadotropin secretion and an impaired response to castration – *i.e.* it has hypogonadotropic hypogonadism (HH)[39]. Weight loss, when forced upon the *ob/ob* mouse by dietary restriction, does not restore fertility. Leptin administration, however, results in a prompt return of fertility, presumably through stimulation of GnRH[40] released. Indeed, leptin-treated *ob/ob* mice have higher serum concentrations released of LH (particularly in females) and FSH (particularly in males) compared with pair-fed saline-treated *ob/ob* mice[41].

Human counterparts of the ob and db (leptin resistant) mice have recently been reported. A missense mutation, identical to the C->T transition in the first base of codon 15 that leads to the appearance of the premature stop codon in the *ob/ob* mouse, has been described in a Turkish kindred[14]. The mutation impaired normal processing of leptin through the secretory pathway. The phenotype of homozygous adults (low serum leptin concentrations associated with hyperphagic obesity and hypothalamic HH) suggests that in humans too, leptin not only controls body mass but is also necessary for the initiation of puberty. More widespread pituitary dysfunction was observed in patients homozygous for a mutation in the gene encoding the leptin receptor[15]. In this consanguineous family, a GA base substitution in the splice donor site of exon 16 resulted in a truncated leptin receptor that lacked both transmembrane and intracellular domains, Affected individuals had very raised serum leptin concentrations together with a history of early onset morbid obesity and lack of pubertal development. In addition there was reduced secretion of growth hormone (causing a mild but significant delay in growth) and thyrotropin (causing mild hypothalamic hypothyroidism).

Women with subnormal body weight, for example those with anorexia nervosa, are hypoleptinaemic[34]. Although the results of treatment of such patients with recombinant leptin have not (yet) been reported, for the reasons set out above it is most likely that the reproductive disturbance results from the leptin deficiency. Characteristically these patients have extremely low levels of LH although serum FSH concentrations are relatively maintained. There is a reduction in LH pulse amplitude and some reduction in pulse frequency[42]. Absent ovarian follicular activity results in subnormal oestradiol secretion. As a result of subnormal LH stimulation, androgen secretion by theca cells is reduced and less testosterone than normal is available for aromatisation, both within and outside the ovary. Moreover, the loss of adipose tissue means that extra glandular aromatisation of adrenal androgens is reduced. Finally, thin women metabolise oestrogens preferentially by 2-rather than by 16-hydroxylation of oestrone, that is to say, by formation of the catechol anti oestrogen, 2-hydroxy oestrone, rather than oestriol[43].

Measurement of serum gonadotrophin concentrations before and during treatment provides information of considerable interest. As body weight approaches normal – and ovulatory menstrual cycles develop without medical treatment – the serum LH returns into the normal range. The answer to the patient's question about her optimal weight is therefore that it is that weight which is associated with a return of pituitary hormone secretion to normal. In our experience this answer is intuitively acceptable to the patient who has had the role of leptin explained. The weight is usually that which produces a body mass index above 19.5 kg/m^2 although the particular weight and body mass index will depend on the patient's level of physical exercise and inter-individual variation. Comparison of 22 women with hypothalamic amenorrhoea with eumenorrhoeic controls, matched for age, BMI (20.6+-1.3 vs 21.1+-1.5 kg/m^2) and fat mass, revealed significantly lower plasma leptin concentrations in the amenorrhoeic group (6.9+-2.9 vs 10.6+-4.9). The amenorrhoiec women ingested significantly less fat, despite having very similar total energy intake to the eumenorrhoiec controls[44].

Some years ago we measured serum gonadotrophin concentrations during the follicular and luteal phases of women undergoing induction of ovulation with pulsatile GnRH[45]. It is necessary here to draw attention to a similar study published some years later by the Bologna group[46], but to emphasise two crucial differences in study design. The first is in the selection, or perhaps more precisely, in the classification of the patients studied and the second is the dose and route of administration of GnRH. The Bologna group used doses of 2.5 and 5 micrograms given intravenously every 60 minutes. We used

15 micrograms given subcutaneously every 90 minutes. In our study we found that, for all diagnostic groups of patients, mean follicular phase serum FSH concentrations were indistinguishable (about 5 mIU/L) in cycles in which ovulation was inferred from a normal serum progesterone concentration in the luteal phase, or proven by the occurrence of pregnancy. In contrast, serum LH concentrations varied hugely according to diagnostic group, being very high in women with PCOS, intermediate in those with IHH and significantly lower in those with weight related amenorrhoea and persistently subnormal weight. This variation was independent of treatment and was observed in ovulatory cycles. We had noted an association of miscarriage with high follicular phase LH levels[47], but were unable to associate any significant biological effect of the remarkably subnormal LH concentrations in the follicular phase of the women with weight related amenorrhoea.

Conclusions

We conclude that considerable heterogeneity exists with respect to gonadotropin secretion in women with HH, both before and during treatment. This is partly related to the aetiology of HH, for example the selective suppression of LH in weight loss related amenorrhoea compared with the reduction in both LH and FSH in subjects with Kallmann's syndrome. However, there is also heterogeneity to be found within a diagnostic grouping, for example the increasing LH secretion as weight is regained, the late failure of gonadotropin secretion in adult onset HH, and our own observations on the recovery of gonadotropin secretion in some patients with phenotypical Kallmann's syndrome. The use of recombinant monohormonal gonadotropin preparations for ovulation-induction in HH, potentially amplifies the importance of background, endogenous gonadotropin secretion in a given treatment cycle. Recognition of this inter-individual and inter-group variability may entail developing bespoke, rather than off-the-peg treatment paradigms in the future.

References

1. Naftolin F., Harris G.W., Bobrow M.: Effect of purified luteinizing hormone releasing factor on normal and hypogonadotrophic anosmic men. *Nature,* 232:496-497, 1971.
2. Yoshimoto Y., Moridera K., Imura H.: Restoration of normal pituitary gonadotropin reserve by administration of luteinizing-hormone-releasing hormone in patients with hypogonadotropic hypogonadism. *N. Engl. J. Med.,* 292:242-245, 1975.

3. Habiby R.L., Boepple P.A., Nachtigall L.B., et al.: Adrenal hypoplasia congenita with hypogonadotropic hypogonadism: evidence that DAX-1 mutations lead to combined hypothalamic and pituitary defects in gonadotropin production. *J. Clin. Invest.*, 98:1055-1062, 1996.
4. de Roux N., Young J., Misrahi M., et al.: A family with hypogonadotropic hypogonadism and mutations in the gonadotropin-releasing hormone receptor. *N. Engl. J. Med.*, 337:1597-602, 1997.
5. Layman L.C., Cohen D.P., Jin M., et al.: Mutations in gonadotropin-releasing hormone receptor gene cause hypogonadotropic hypogonadism. *Nature. Genet.*, 18:14-15, 1998.
6. Forest M.G., Cathiard A.M., Bertrand J.A.: Total and unbound testosterone levels in the newborn and in normal and hypogonadal children: use of a sensitive radioimmunoassay for testosterone. *J. Clin. Endocrinol. Metab.*, 36:1132-1142, 1973.
7. de Zegher, Devlieger H., Veldhuis J.D.: Pulsatile and sexually dimorphic secretion of luteinizing hormone in the human infant on the day of birth. *Pediatr. Res.*, 32:605-607, 1992.
8. Spratt D.I., Carr D.B., Merriam G.R., et al.: The spectrum of abnormal patterns of gonadotropin-releasing hormone secretion in men with idiopathic hypogonadotropic hypogonadism: clinical and laboratory correlations. *J. Clin. Endocrinol. Metab.*, 64:283-291, 1987.
9. Weiss J., Crowley W.F., Jr., Jameson J.L.: Normal structure of the gonadotropin-releasing hormone (GnRH) gene in patients with GnRH deficiency and idiopathic hypogonadotropic hypogonadism. *J. Clin. Endocrinol. Metab.*, 69:299-303, 1989.
10. Franco B., Guioli S., Pragliola A., et al.: A gene deleted in Kallmann's syndrome shares homology with neural cell adhesion and axonal path finding molecules. *Nature*, 353:529-535, 1991.
11. Legouis R., Hardelin J.-P., Levilliers J., et al.: The candidate gene for the X-linked Kallmann syndrome encodes a protein related to adhesion molecules. *Cell*, 67:423-435, 1991.
12. Zanaria E., Muscatelli F., Bardoni B., et al.: An unusual member of the nuclear hormone receptor superfamily responsible for X-linked adrenal hypoplasia congenita. *Nature*, 372:635-641, 1994.
13. Muscatelli F., Strom T.M., Walker A.P., et al.: Mutations in the DAX-1 gene give rise to both X-linked adrenal hypoplasia congenita and hypogonadotropic hypogonadism. *Nature*, 372:672-676, 1994.
14. Strobel A., Issad T., Camoin L., et al.: A leptin missense mutation associated with hypogonadism and morbid obesity. *Nature Genet.*, 18:213-215, 1998.

15. Clement K., Vaisse C., Lahlou N., et al.: A mutation in the human leptin receptor gene causes obesity and pituitary dysfunction. *Nature,* 392:398-401, 1998.
16. Jackson R.S., Creemers J.W., Ohagi S., et al.: Obesity and impaired prohormone processing associated with mutations in the human prohormone convertase 1 gene [see comments]. *Nature Genet.,* 16:303-6, 1997.
17. Holmes G.: A form of familial degeneration of the cerebellum. *Brain,* 30:466-489, 1907.
18. Berciano J., Amado J.A., Freijanes J., et al.: Familial cerebellar ataxia and hypogonadotropic hypogonadism: evidence for hypothalamic LHRH deficiency. *J. Neurol. Neurosurg. Psychiat.,* 45:747-751, 1995.
19. Dattani M.T., Martinez-Barbera J.-P., Thomas P.Q., et al.: Mutations in the homeobox gene HESX1/Hesx1 associated with septo-optic dysplasia in human and mouse. *Nature Genet.,* 19:125-133, 1998.
20. Quinton R., Conway G.S., Vanderpump M.P.J., et al.: Adult-onset idiopathic hypogonadotrophic hypogonadism may be over-diagnosed. *B.M.J.,* 317:600-601, 1998.
21. Puig-Domingo-M., Webb S.M., Serrano J., et al.: Brief report: melatonin-related hypogonadotropic hypogonadism [see comments]. *N. Engl. J. Med.,* 327:1356-1359, 1992.
22. Walker A.B., English J., Arendt J., et al.: Hypogonadotrophic hypogonadism and primary amenorrhoea associated with increased melatonin secretion from a cystic pineal lesion. *Clin. Endocrinol.* Oxf., 45:353-356, 1996.
23. Schwanzel-Fukuda M., Pfaff D.W.: Origin of luteinizing hormone-releasing hormone neurons. *Nature,* 338:161-164, 1989.
24. Schwanzel-Fukuda M., Bick D.P., Pfaff D.W.: Luteinizing hormone-releasing hormone (LHRH)-expressing cells do not migrate normally in an inherited hypogonadal (Kallmann) syndrome. *Mol. Brain Res,* 6:311-326.
25. Georgopoulos N.A., Pralong F.P., Seidman C.E., et al.: Genetic heterogeneity evidenced by low incidence of KAL-1 gene mutations in sporadic cases of gonadotropin-releasing hormone deficiency. *J. Clin. Endocrinol. Metab.,* 82:213-217, 1997.
26. Quinton R., Kirk J.M.W., Matfin G., et al.: *Phenotypic aspects of isolated GnRH deficiency in males.* Endocrine Society Annual Congress. New Orleans, pp. 2-46, 1998.
27. Fromantin M., Grieste J., Didier A., Ronnier J.: Les impuberisms et les hypogonadisms a l'incorporation. *Probl. Act. Endocrinol. Nutr.,* 16:179-199, 1972.
28. Jones J.R., Kemmann E.: Olfacto-genital dysplasia in the female. *Obstet. Gynecol. Annu.,* 5:443-466, 1976.

29. Nachtigall L.B., Boepple P.A., Pralong F.P., Crowley W.F., Jr.: Adult-onset idiopathic hypogonadotropic hypogonadism -a treatable form of male infertility. *N. Engl. J. Med.*, 336:410-415, 1997.
30. Quinton R., Cheow H.K., Bouloux P.-M.G., et al.: Kallmann's syndrome: is it always for life? *Clin. Endocrinol.* Oxf., (in press).
31. van der Spuy S., Steer P.J., McCusker M., et al.: Outcome of pregnancy in underweight women after spontaneous and induced ovulation. *B.M.J.*, 296:962-965, 1988.
32. Dennison E., Fall C., Cooper C., Barker D.: Prenatal factors influencing long-term outcome. *Hormone Res.*, 48(Suppl 1):25-9, 1997.
33. Aakvaag A., Sand T., Opstad P.K., Fonnum-F.: Hormonal changes in serum in young men during prolonged physical strain. *Eur. J. Appl. Physiol.*, 39:283-91, 1978.
34. Conway G.S., Jacobs H.S.: Leptin: a hormone of reproduction. *Hum. Reprod.*, 12:633- 635, 1997.
35. Stephens T.W., Basinski M., Bristow P.K., et al.: The role of neuropeptide Y in the antiobesity action of the obese gene product. *Nature*, 377:530-532, 1995.
36. Stephens T.W.: Life without neuropeptide Y. *Nature*, 381:377-378, 1998.
37. Erickson J.C., Ahima R.S., Hollopeter G., et al.: Endocrine function of neuropeptide Y knockout mice. *Regulatory Peptides*, 70:199-202, 1997.
38. Friedman J.M.: The alphabet of weight control. *Nature*, 385:119-120, 1998.
39. Swerdloff R.S., Batt R.A., Bray G.A.: Reproductive hormonal function in the genetically obese (*ob/ob*) mouse. *Endocrinology*, 98:1359-64,1976.
40. Chehab F.F., Lim M.E., Lu R.: Correction of the sterility defect in homozygous obese female mice by treatment with the human recombinant leptin. *Nature Genet.*, 12(3):318-320, 1996.
41. Barash I.A., Cheung C.C., Weigle D.S., et al.: Leptin is a metabolic signal to the reproductive system. *Endocrinology*, 137:3144-3147, 1996.
42. Berga S.L., Mortola J.F., Girton L., et al.: Neuroendocrine aberrations in women with functional hypothalamic amenorrhea. *J. Clin. Endocrinol. Metab.*, 68:301-308, 1989.
43. Balen A.H., Shoham Z., Jacobs H.S.: Amenorrhoea -causes and consequences In: Asch R.H., Studd J.W.W. (eds). *Annual Progress in Reproductive Medicine.* Parthenon, New York, pp 205-234, 1993.
44. Miller K., Parulekar M., Schoenfeld E., et al.: *Hypoleptinaemia in women with hypothalamic amenorrhoeia.* Endocrine Society Annual Congress. New Orleans: OR13-3, 1998.
45. Abdulwahid N.A., Adams J., van der Spuy S., Jacobs H.S.: Gonadotrophin control of follicular development. *Clin. Endocrinol.* Oxf., 23: 613-626, 1985.

46. Filicori M., Flamigni C., Meriggiola M.C., et al.: Endocrine response determines the clinical outcome of pulsatile gonadotropin-releasing hormone ovulation induction in different ovulatory disorders. *J. Clin. Endocrinol. Metab.*, 72:965-972, 1991.
47. Balen A.H., Tan S.L., Jacobs H.S.: Hypersecretion of luteinising hormone: a significant cause of infertility and miscarriage. *Brit. J. Obstet. Gynaecol.*, 100:1082-1089, 1993

The Role of Luteinizing Hormone
in Folliculogenesis
and Ovulation Induction, pp. 105-114
Editor M. Filicori

Effects of Different Menotropin Preparations for Ovulation Induction in Hypogonadotropic Women

Z. Shoham

Department of Obstetrics and Gynecology
Kaplan Medical Center, Rehovot (Israel)

Abstract. *The relative importance of LH in the follicular phase and its role in the stimulation of the follicle is uncertain, and the optimal amount of LH or the ratio of FSH:LH in the gonadotropin preparation used remains a problem that dates back to the early days of gonadotropin therapy. Preliminary evidence suggested that preparations that exhibited remarkable differences in FSH:LH ratio of more than 10-fold did not interfere with the clinical efficacy, provided a large enough dose of FSH was given. In patients with hypogonadotropic amenorrhea, Berger and Taymor demonstrated that treatment with pituitary FSH alone did not result in follicular* E_2 *secretion and had therefore concluded that LH was essential for ovulation induction. Looking at the results of induction of ovulation in 9 hypogonadotropic patients, using uFSH vs hMG it was found that the follicular phase was longer (22.3 ± 7.6 vs. 17.6 ± 5.4 days, respectively,* $p<0.02$*) total number of ampoules was higher (27.6 ± 16.9 vs. 35.3 ± 21.7, respectively,* $p<0.004$*) more follicles of* $\geq$ *16 mm in diameter had developed (2.0 ± 0.7 vs. 1.2 ± 0.4, respectively,* $P<0.05$*) and serum* E_2 *concentration on the day of hCG was higher (1477 ± 985 pg/mL vs. 377 ± 299 pg/mL, respectively,* $p<0.002$*). Ovulation was achieved in only 33% of patients treated with uFSH. The use of r-hFSH in hypogonadotropic patients up to a dose of 3,150 IU showed a maximum of* E_2 *serum levels of 139.5 pmol/L, at the time of maximum follicular growth. At that time mean concentrations of serum LH, A, and T (0.11 IU/L, 2.2 nmol/L, and 0.48 nmol/L, respectively) were comparable with those measured at baseline. Serum P was undetectable during treatment and no change in endometrial thickness was observed. In a prospective, randomized, dose-finding study using a fixed dose of r-hFSH (150 IU) and increased doses of r-hLH (from placebo to 225 IU) the efficacy of r-hLH for supporting r-hFSH was investigated in 38 hypogonadotropic women. Recombinant-hLH was found to promote dose-related increases in* E_2 *secretion, increase the ovarian sensitivity to FSH, and enhance the ability of these follicles to luteinize when exposed to hCG. A daily dose of 75 IU r-hLH was found to be effective in the majority of women in promoting optimal* *follicular development (defined as ≥ 1 follicle ≥ 17 mm; E_2 ≥ 400 pmol/L; mid-luteal phase P ≥ 25 nmol/L and maximal endometrial growth. A minority of patients may require up to 225 IU/day. These findings and those of others support the notion that normal follicular development is dependent predominantly on FSH and that steroidogenesis is mainly supported by the synergistic action of FSH and LH.*

Key words. Hypogonadotropic hypogonadism, ovulation induction, follicular development, Human Menopausal gonadotropin, recombinant follicle stimulation hormone, recombinant luteinizing hormone.

Introduction

There is no doubt that morphological and functional changes occurring within the follicle during the preovulatory period are of primary importance for final maturation of the ovum. It has, however, become increasingly apparent that hormonal events before the midcycle LH peak, specifically the fluctuation of LH and FSH during the early follicular phase, may significantly influence the development of the oocyte and determine its subsequent meiotic capability and fertilization ability.

The importance of pituitary FSH in control of ovarian function during the follicular phase is beyond question. FSH plays a major role in female reproduction, by stimulating gonadal differentiation and maturation via its regulatory action on the granulosa cell in the ovary[1]. Studies in rodents show that, during the follicular phase, FSH controls major morphological and cellular events such as acquisition of the antral cavity, induction or activation of enzymes involved in progesterone biosynthesis, induction of luteinizing hormone (LH) receptors on granulosa cells, and, in combination with androgens produced by the theca under LH control, FSH induces or activates the aromatase system, which enables the follicle to produce estrogen, to ovulate and luteituze in response to the gonadotropin surge[2]. The relative importance of LH in the follicular phase and its role in the stimulation of the follicle is uncertain and the optimal amount of LH, or the ratio of FSH: LH in the stimulating drugs used, is a problem that dates back to the early days of gonadotropin therapy[3].

Patients with hypogonadotropic hypogonadism have a clinical syndrome that results from impairment of neuroendocrine function and presents with amenorrhea and small ovaries with arrested fulliculogenesis. Therefore, in order to investigate the physiology of the gonadotropin actions regarding steroidogenesis and follicular development, and to explore the minimal effective dose of FSH and LH needed, patients with hypogonadotropic hypogonadism can serves as the best model for this physiological investigations.

Historical Overview

The theory that both gonadotropins are required for complete stimulation of follicular maturation dates back fifty years. Fevold[4] was the first to point out, in 1941, that treatment with highly purified FSH increased ovarian growth and follicle development in immature hypophysectomized rats without stimulating the release of estrogen. A year later, Greep et al.[5] demonstrated in hypophysectomized rats that FSH resulted in follicular growth only and that whole pituitary extract, with presumed LH activity, was necessary to produce uterine growth indicating follicular production of estrogen. Additional data were obtained by Short[6] and Ryan et al.[7] who demonstrated that while both theca and granulosa cells had the capacity to synthesize steroids in vitro, the production of estradiol by granulosa cells was markedly enhanced by the addition of theca cells.

In 1959, Falck[8], in his thesis presented at the university of Lund, and entitled "Site of the production of estrogen in rat ovary as studies in Microtransplants" gave rise to the two-cell theory. In an elegant study, he provided the first evidence that ovarian estrogen biosynthesis required the interplay of at least two ovarian cell types. He isolated granulosa, theca, interstitial, and luteal cells and autotransplanted these cell types either alone or in combination to the eye chamber of spayed female rats. The results indicated that estrogen was produced only when theca or interstitial cells were co-transplanted with granulosa cells or luteal cells or when intact follicles were autotransplanted. These results also emphasized the critical interplay between LH and FSH for normal estradiol production.

Later on, Eshkol and Lunenfeld[9] in rodents and Berger and Taymor[10] in patients with hypogonadotropic amenorrhea demonstrated that treatment with pituitary FSH alone did not result in follicular estrogen secretion and concluded that LH was essential for final follicular maturation and ovulation induction. These observations gave additional support to the two-cell, two-gonadotropin theory of follicular steroidogenesis. According to this hypothesis the ovarian theca cells stimulated by LH secrete androgens that transverse through the basal membrane into the granulosa cells where the FSH-augmented excessive enzyme system turns them into estrogen[6,7]. Thus the synergistic action of both gonadotropins is presumed to be necessary for follicular maturation and steroidogenesis. However, not everyone agreed with this notion. It was Kenigsberg and his colleagues[11] who showed that in monkeys rendered hypogonadotropic by the administration of GnRH antagonists, injecting increased doses of purified urinary FSH caused multiple follicular development, and ovulation could apparently be induced by the administration of hCG. This theory received some support from studies of ovulation induction and IVF programs, using GnRH agonist for pitutary desensitization, because the fertilization rate after oocyte retrieval was similar with urinary FSH or urinary hMG preparations, the latter containing considerable amounts of LH activity. Thus, it might be possible that remaining endogenous LH during GnRH suppression seems to he sufficient for follicular maturation[12].

Clinical Data

Following the development of urofollitrophin FSH (FSH, Metrodin) it was found that FSH alone administered in pharmacological doses, to women who do not secrete FSH and LH, i.e. women with hypogonadotropic hypogonadism, caused follicular development similar to that achieved with hMG. However, only a few of these women ovulated in response to hCG administration[13,14]. Shoham et al.[13] gave treatment to patients with hypogonadotropic hypogonadism during consecutice cycles, using the same stimulation protocol, with hMG in the first treatment cycle and urinary FSH in the second one. Compared with hMG, treatment with urinary FSH required significantly more ampules of drug ($p<0.04$) but resulted in a significant reduction in the number of leading follicles ($p<0.05$), serum estradiol concentrations ($p<0.002$), endometrial thickness ($p<0.02$) and the occurrence of ovulation ($p<0.05$) (Table 1). This study showed that in patients with hypogonadotropic hypogonadism the superior efficacy of hMG compared with urinary FSH preparation is beyond question. This phenomenon may have been related to the inadequate estradiol secretion following this mode of treatment.

The above mentioned observation raised the immediate question of how much LH is needed during the follicular phase, in order to maintain estrogen production and an appropriate endometrial development. To answer this question Shoham and his colleagues[15] designed a study, in two patients with isolated hypogonadotropic hypogonadism, to examine ovarian performance, i,e, follicular growth, normal steroidogenesis and luteal phase function, following the administration of multiple increasing doses of urinary FSH with a constant low dose of LH. HMG was used in the first treatment cycle, starting with 150 IU of LH and 150 IU of FSH per day, for 7 days. The dose was increased daily with 75 IU of LH and 75 IU of FSH for another 7 days if no response was detected by serial ultrasound measurements and serum estradiol determinations. In the second treatment cycle, a constant dose of 75 IU of LH (using hMG) was administered per day and up to 150 IU of FSH (using urofollitrophin) was supplemented. If no response was detected after 7 days of treatment, the dose of FSH was increased. For the final stage of oinduction,

TABLE 1 - *Clinical and Laboratory results of hMG/urinary FSH treatment cycles in 9 patients with hypogonadotropic hypogonadism.*

Patients No.	*Days of Treatment*	*No. of Amps. Used*	*Follicles >16mm*	*E2 on hCG day (Pmol/L)*	*Endometrial thickness (mm)*	*Midluteal Progesterone (nmol/L)*
1	14/16	17/20	2/1	2300/236	8/5	51/<2
2	28/32	60/72	1/2	497/246	7/5	17/<2
3	16/25	24/32	3/1	3060/240	9/5	>100/<2
4	10/18	12/16	2/1	1384/739	9/9	>100/>100
5	14/16	14/16	1/1	540/477	9/5	48/77
6	18/19	22/31	3/1	1212/183	10/7	50/<2
7	20/22	31/36	2/2	1130/134	9/5	>100/>100
8	14/16	18/21	2/1	460/153	10/7	67/7
9	23/37	51/71	2/1	2710/987	8/8	42/<2
Mean	17.6/22.3	27.6/35.3	2.0/1.2	1477/377	8.7/6.2	
± SD	5.4/7.6	16.9/21.7	0.7/0.4	985/299	1.0/1.5	
P	<0.02	<0.004	<0.05	<0.002	<0.02	

hCG was administered in the presence of at least one follicle >17 mm in diameter but with no more than three follicles >16 mm in diameter. To verify the adequacy of the luteal phase, a pharmacokinetic/pharmacodynamic study of HCG, estradiol and progesterone was performed following the second treatment cycle only. It was found that ovarian stimulation using a constant dose of 75 IU of LH and increasing doses of FSH up to 225 IU, resulted in normal follicular growth and hormonal milieu. Both women showed normal luteal phase estradiol and progesterone production and both women conceived following the second treatment cycle.

Recently, following the development of recombinant human FSH, which is completely devoid of LH activity, Mannaerts and her colleagues[16] in an elegant study in immature hypophysectomized female rats, showed that treatment with recombinant FSH increased ovarian weight and aromatase activity in a ose-dependent manner. However, when recombinant FSH doses providing submaximal responses were subsequently supplemented with 1 IU of hCG (as an LH substitute), both ovarian weight and aromatase activity were greatly augmented. In this study, the authors also showed that recombinant FSH alone is unable to increase circulating estradiol, while a combination of FSH and 0.1 IU hCG provided a 3-fold increase in median plasma estradiol levels. This study indicates that LH, although not obligatory for stimulating follicular growth, is necessary for stimulating adequate follicular function (Table 2).

The possibility of examining the physiology and the role of FSH in ovulation induction became available when the recombinant FSH was available for clinical use. In a study conducted by Shoham et al.[17] 2 women with hypogonadotropic hypogonadism volunteered to receive treatment with increasing doses of recombinant FSH (Org 32489; Organon International, Oss, The Netherlands). The results in this report are part of a multicenter study that was conducted to examine pharmacokinetics, pharmacodynamics, safety, and tolerance of a recombinant human FSH preparation devoid of LH activity. This study was an open phase I multiple rising dose study. The drug was administered intramuscularly one time per day for a maximum 21 days, i.e. 75 IU for the first 7 days, 150 IU for the next 7 days, and 225 IU during the last 7 days. Treatment was discontinue if serum estradiol was $\geq$ 1100 pmol/L and or one or more growing follicle >14 mm in diameter was observed. It was found that treatment with recombinant FSH resulted in dose-related increase of serum FSH. Both women showed follicular growth, whereas serum androstendione concentrations were very low, and serum estradiol concentrations rose to only 76.7 and 139.5 pmol/L respectively. This study support the theory of the two-cell two gonadotropin, that FSH alone can induce follicular growth. The low concentrations of androstendione and estradiol indicate the need for

TABLE 2 - *Hypophysectomized rates were treated with different doses of recombinanr FSH and with increasing doses of hCG. In the absence of hCG, or with 40 IU of recombinant FSH no significant increase in plasma estradiol was noted. When 1 IU of hCG was addedd to the recombinant FSH serum plasma estradiol was increase in a dose dependent manner.* (Summariesed from Mannaerts et al. Endocrinology 129:2623-2630, 1991).

Treatment	*Total dose (IU) FSH*	*Total dose (IU) hCG*	*Estradiol (pg/ml)*
Recombinant FSH	0	None	8.9
	5	None	10.4
	10	None	9.6
	20	None	10.0
	40	None	10.8
Recombinant FSH and hCG	0	1	3.6
	5	1	93.8
	10	1	95.7
	20	1	200
	40	1	454
Recombinant FSH and hCG	40	0	10.9
	40	0.1	34.3
	40	1	674
	40	10	1090
	40	40	1440

LH to induce appropriate steroidogenesis.

In a very recent publication[18] by the Recombinant Human LH Study Group, the efficacy of recombinant human luteinizing hormone (r-hLH) and human-follicle stimulating hormone (r-hFSH)-induced were investigated in hypogonadotropic hypogonadal women. The aim of this clinical study with recombinant LH was to determine the minimal effective dose of LH needed for the support of FSH to induce follicular development in LH and FSH deficient anovulatory women with hypogonadotropic hypogonadism. Patients (n=38, 18 with primary and 10 with secondary hypogonadism) were randomized to receive r-hLH, 0, 25, 75 or 225 IU/day (Lhadi, Ares-Serono, Switzerland) in addition to a fixed dose of r-hFSH (Gonal-F, Ares-Serono, Switzerland), 150 IU/day. Ovulation was induced with the administration of 10,000 IU of hCG, when at least one follicle reached a diameter of ≥ 17 mm and there was no risk of developing OHSS. The results of this report will relate to the first cycle only since in this cycle treatment with recombinant LH was randomized between patients. The efficacy end points were: one follicle with a mean diameter of >17 mm, a preovulatory serum estradiol level of > 400 pmol/L and mid-luteal phase progesterone level >25 nmol/L. In the first treatment cycle 10 patients were treated with 225 IU, 9 were treated with 75 IU, 7 were treated with 25 IU and 8 were treated with O IU (placebo) of r-hLH. Out of the 19 patients receiving r-hLH, 75 IU or 225 IU once daily 15 had follicular growth by contrast to those receiving 0 or 25 IU of r-hLH since only 4 patients had excessive follicular growth. Because the dose of r-hFSH was fixed and identical for all patients, this strongly suggests that r-hLH enhances the ovarian response to FSH.

Out of the 38 patients 17 patients received hCG, 5 did not receive hCG because of the risk of OHSS, 14 did not receive hCG because of insufficient follicular development and 2 withdrew consent. A significant relationship (P=0.0210) was observed between the dose of r-hLH and the percentage of patients achieving optimal steroidogenesis, defined as estradiol > 400 pmol/L and P, > 25 nmol/L. In addition, dose-related effect of r-hLH on follicular development was noted. During the follicular phase, there was a clear relationship between the dose of r-hLH and serum estradiol, with the highest levels recorded in patients treated with 225 IU/day and the lowest among those receiving O IU/day. The difference in serum estradiol concentrations between the groups not only reflects a difference in the number of growing follicles but results from a very significant difference in output of estradiol per follicles > 15 mm. Endometrial growth was similar and optimal in both the 75 IU and the 225 IU r-hLH treatment groups, even though serum estradiol concentrations were twice as high in the 225 IU group.

Conclusions

In patients with hypogonadotropic hypogonadism, FSH is required for follicular growth, however, some LH is necessary to achieve adequate steroidogenesis and develop follicle capacity to ovulate and luteinized when exposed to hCG. When FSH alone is used to stimulate follicular development, follicular growth occurs but estradiol concentrations is minimal leading to insufficient endometrial growth. It seems as if the majority of patients suffering from hypogonadotropic hypogonadism receiving 75 IU/day of recombinant LH will respond adequately.

References

1. Hsueh A.J., Adashi E.Y., Jones P., Welsh T.H. Jr.: Hormonal regulation of the differentiation of cultured ovanan granulosa cells. *Endocrinol. Rev.*, 5: 76-127, 1984.

2. Zeleznik A.J., Hillier S.C.: The role of gonadotropins in the selection of the preovulatory follicle. *Clin. Obstet. Gynecol.*, 27:927-940, 1984.
3. Jacobson A., Marshall J.R.: Ovulatory response rate with human menopausal gonadotropins of varying FSH/LH ratios. *Fertil. Steril.*, 20:171-173, 1984.
4. Fevold H.L.: Synergism of follicle stimulating and Luteinizing hormones in producing estrogen secretion. *Endocrinology*, 28:33-6, 1941.
5. Greep R.O., van Dyke H.E., Chow B.F.: Gonadotropin of swine pituitary: various biological effects of purified thylkentrin (FSH) and pure matakentrin (ICSH). *Endocrinology*, 30:635-649, 1942.
6. Short R.V.: Steroids in the follicular fluid and the corpus luteum of the mare. A "two-cell type" theory of ovarian steroid synthesis. *J. Endocrinol.*, 24:59-63, 1962.
7. Ryan K.J., Petro Z., Kaiser J.: Steroid formation by isolated and recombined ovarian granulosa and theca cells. *J. Clin. Endocrinol. Metab.*, 28:355-358, 1968.
8. Falk B.: Site of production of oestrogen in rat ovary as studied in microtransplants. *Acta Physiol. Scand.*, 47(Suppl)163:1-101, 1959.
9. Eshkol A., Lunenfeld B.: Purification and separation of follicle-stimulating hormone (FSH) and luteinizing hormone (LH) from human menopausal gonadotropin (HMG). *Acta Endocrinol.* (Copenh), 54:91-95, 1967.
10. Berger M.J., Taymor M.L.: The role of luteinizing hormone in human follicular maturation function. *Am. J. Obstet. Gynecol.*, 111:708-710, 1971.
11. Kenigsberg D., Littman B.A., Williams R.F., Hodgen G.D.: Mechanical hypophysectomy. II. Variability of ovarian responsiveness to gonadotropin therapy. *Fertil. Steril.*, 42:116-126, 1984.
12. Bentick R., Shaw R.W., Iffland C.A., Burfard G., Bernard: Randomized comparative study of purified follicle stimulating hormone and human menopausal gonadotropin after pituitary desensitization with buserelin for superovulation and in vitro fertilization. *Fertil. Steril.*, 50:79-84, 1988.
13. Shoham Z., Balen A., Patel A., Hacobs H.S.: Results of ovulation induction using human menopausal gonadotropin or purified follicle-stimulating hormone in hypogonadotropic hypogonadism patients. *Fertil. Steril.*, 56:1048-1053, 1991.
14. Couzinet B., Lestart N., Brailly S., Forest M., Schaison G.: Stimulation of ovarian follicle maturation with purefollicle-stimulating hormone in women with gonadotropin deficiency. *J. Clin. Endocrinol. Metab.*, 66:552-556;1988.
15. Shoham Z., Howles C.M., Zalel Y., Weissman A., Insler V.: Induction of follicular growth and production of a normal hormonal milieu in spite of using a constant low dose of luteinizing hormone in women with hypog-

onadotropic hypogonadism. *Hum. Reprod.*, 9:431-436, 1994.

16. Mannaerts B., de Leeuw R., Geelen J., Van Ravestein A., Wezenbeek P.V.I., Schuurs A.: Comparative in vitro and in vive studies on the biological characteristics of recombinant human follicle stimulating hormone. *Endocrinology*, 129:2623-2630, 1991.
17. Shoham Z., Mannaerts B., Insler V., Coeling-Bennink H.J.: Induction of follicular growth using recombinant human follicle-stimulating hormone in two volunteer women with hypogonadotropic hypogonadism. *Fertil. Steril.*, 59:738-742, 1993.
18. Recombinant Human LH Study Group: Recombinant human luteinizing hormone (r-hLH) to support recombinant human follicle stimulating hormone (r-hFSH)-induced follicular development in LH and FSH deficient anovulatory women: a dose-finding study. *J. Clin. Endoc. Metabol.*, 83:1507-1514, 1998.

The Role of Luteinizing Hormone
in Folliculogenesis
and Ovulation Induction, pp. 115-133
Editor M. Filicori

Pathogenesis of Anovulation in Polycystic Ovary Syndrome

A. Lanzone, M. Ciampelli, A.M. Fulghesu, F. Cucinelli, G. Muzj, E. Pierro, M. Guido, L. Soranna, C. Belosi, C. Perri and F. Serri*

Department of Obstetrics and Gynecology
Università Cattolica del Sacro Cuore, Rome (Italy)
** Department of Obstetrics and Gynecology, University of Cagliari (Italy)*

Abstract. *Polycystic ovary syndrome (PCOS) is an endocrine disorder that compromises normal follicular development. Folliculogenesis is lacking in the ovaries of these patients, which arrest the normal recruitment and selection of dominant preovulatory follicles. The initial steps of folliculogenesis seem intact in PCOS, although the subsequesnt steps are defective; the exact mechanisms underlying this phenomenon are unknown, even if many suggestions indicate gonadotropins as a main factor in the pathogenesis of anovulation in this syndrome. It has been postulated that the elevated circulating luteinizing hormone (LH) concentration by itself or, subsequently, the intraovarian hyperandrogenism, may produce an inadequate follicle stimulating hormone (FSH) induced estrogen response, which in turn may compromise the maturation of the developing follicle, thereby creating a cohort of small antral follicles.*

On the other hand recent data suggested that elevated insulin levels might contribute to the mechanisms of anovulation by interacting with and/or increasing LH. It becomes so clear the influence of the metabolic status of such anovulatory patients on the ovarian function regulation; the prevalence of obesity in PCOS is rather high, ranging from 30 to 60% whereas an exaggerated insulin response to glucose load associated with insulin resistance is present in more than 50% of PCOS patients. Furthermore, although about 70% of obese PCOS women exhibited hyperinsulinemia, this feature is also present in 20-40% of lean subjects. Recently some investigators showed that obesity in PCOS is associated with an attenuation of LH pulse amplitude and LH response to GnRH stimulus, not accounted for obesity per se, but also for insulin resistance, thus arguing against a pathogenetic role of hyperinsulinemia and reduced insulin sensitivity on LH levels in this syndrome. By contrast, other researchers have shown reduced LH levels in conjunction with suppression of insulin levels by insulin lowering drugs in PCOS women, thus suggesting an enhancing influence of insulin on LH secretion. From recent data by our group it could be hypothesized that these conflicting reports might be ascribed to a different impact of hyperinsulinemia in lean and obese patients; in the last ones the main cause of hyperinsulinemia could be represented by reduced peripheral insulin sensitivity, hypothetically present also at the pituitary level. Conversely, in lean patients, hyperinsulinemia, in the absence of related insulin resistance, could act by sensitizing gonadotroph cells.

In any case insulin and related growth factors are able to elicit in vitro the aromatase activity of PCOS granulosa cells to a far greater extent than control granulosa cells, thus suggesting the hypothesis that unspecified factors present in the follicular milieu may block in vivo the aromatase activity, leading to chronic anovulation. This hypothesis seems to be confirmed by recent data showing an involvement of follicular fluid in the pathogenesis of altered steroidal response as well as proliferation rate in granulosa cells from polycystic ovaries. Thus a paracrine control of the ovarian function seem to be highlighted.

In conclusion it could be considered that the mechanisms leading to anovulation in PCOS are very complex in nature and that the metabolic status could constitute a main factor in determining such dysfunction.

Key words. PCOS, insulin, anovulation, LH, FSH, aromatase, growth factors.

Introduction

Polycystic ovary syndrome (PCOS) is the most common cause of anovulatory infertility[1,2], but the mechanism of anovulation remains obscure. Anovulation in PCOS is characterized by an apparent arrest of antral follicle development at the 5-10 mm stage and, therefore, a failure to enter the preovulatory phase of the cycle[3].

Many hypotheses have been made in order to explain this feature; since ovulation can be induced in women with PCOS by the administration of exogenous gonadotropins, it has been suggested that anovulation could be due to a failure of FSH mediated follicular maturation, possibly due to the overproduction of an endocrine or paracrine inhibitor of FSH in women with PCOS[3]. It has been suggested that the elevated circulating LH concentration, which represents a feature of the syndrome, might be responsible, by itself or the subsequent ovarian hyperandrogenism, of the inadequate FSH-stimulated estrogen response[3].

On the other hand recent data suggested that insulin levels might contribute to the mechanisms of anovulation by interacting with and/or increasing LH[4]; considering that an exaggerated insulin response to glucose load associated with insulin resistance is present in more than 50% of PCOS patients, it becomes clear the influence of the metabolic status of such anovulatory patients on the ovarian function regulation.

The purpose of this paper is to discuss the possible mechanisms leading to anovulation in the PCO syndrome.

Role of the hypothalamus

Ovulatory cycles in women result from sequential stimulation of ovarian follicular development by pituitary FSH and LH. In the follicular phase the initial FSH stimulus declines and LH secretion increases toward the mid-cycle ovulatory surge; successively, during the luteal phase, gonadotropin secretion is reduced[5].

The synthesis and the secretion of FSH and LH are regulated by gonadotropin-releasing hormone (GnRH), a peptide which is secreted by the hypothalamus in an intermittent manner with a discharge frequency varying from intervals of 40-60 minutes to 3-5 hours. The frequency of GnRH pulses changes during menstrual cycles, with pulse frequency and amplitude gradually increasing during the follicular phase; following ovulation, pulse frequency slows and remains slow until the demise of the corpus luteum, when frequency again increases to begin the next wave of follicular maturation[5].

Several studies have demonstrated that the frequency and amplitude of LH pulses are increased in patients with PCOS[6,7], though not to supranormal levels. GnRH pulse frequency in PCOS is approximately one pulse per hour, similar to that present during the late follicular phase of ovulatory cycles. Divergent data exist about the presence of hypothalamic disorders at the basis of anovulation in PCOS. Two interesting findings seem to indicate the presence of a primary hypothalamic abnormality in this syndrome; indeed the nocturnal slowing of LH frequency seen in the normal female during the early follicular phase is absent in PCOS[8], which is characterized by a constant frequency troughout the 24h. Furthermore Zumoff and coworkers[9] have reported that in adolescents, LH pulsatility, which is normally exclusively nocturnal in puberty, was delayed 7-8 hours in PCOS.

On the other hand it is important to note that the substances which are capable to modifying gonadotropin function by a direct hypothalamic action (like as clomiphene cytrate) are very effective in PCOS. Moreover it has been demonstrated that the normal action of progesterone in slowing LH pulse frequency is retained in PCOS women[10]. These two last findings seem to argue against a primary hypothalamic abnormality at the basis of anovulation in PCOS patients.

Other researcher have investigated the possibility of an abnormal feedback of gonadal steroids at the hypothalamic levels; indeed it is well known that administration of progesterone during the follicular phase is able to slow GnRH pulse secretion[11], whereas estradiol administration lead to an increase in GnRH pulse frequency and amplitude[12]. Thus it is conceivable that the ovarian hyperandrogenism could be related in PCOS to hypothalamic dysfunction; however, in patients with PCOS, perfusion of testosterone or dihydrotestosterone at plasma levels of normal men has no effect on LH pulsatility or the response to GnRH[13]. Furthermore the administration of a pure non-steroidal antiandrogen to women suffering from PCOS did not show modifications of LH pulsatility, the response to GnRH or the circulating sex steroids levels compared to placebo[5]. It therefore appears that the androgens are not directly responsible for the gonadotrophic disorders; it is more likely that the influence of ovarian hyperandrogenism might be mediated by peripheral aromatization of androgens to estrogens.

Estrone, the major metabolite of androstenedione, is always increased in PCOS; however it does not seem able to influence the pulsatility patterns at the hypothalamic level[14]. On the contrary estradiol is capable of modifying gonadotropin secretion[12], even if plasma levels are not increased in PCOS; considering that PCOS is also characterized by a reduction of Sex Hormone Binding Globulin (SHBG) plasma concentrations, it could be hypothesized that the higher circulating levels of unbound estradiol could be responsible of the hypothalamic disorders of PCOS.

On the other hand the administration of small doses of estradiol to PCOS women does not modify LH frequency, but increases only its amplitude and the response to GnRH[15], thus leading to the hypothesis that two factors might be involved in the pathophysiology of anovulation in PCOS: a primary anomaly of gonadotropin secretion and exacerbation of estradiol positive feedback[15]. However, other factors may be involved, even if it is not possible to disclose whether they have a main role in provoking the disturbance or they are only aggravating factors.

In vitro studies on ovarian steroidogenesis

The traditional view of the function of antral follicles in PCOS is that these represent a largely atretic population, but this is far from the case. Follicular fluid steroids levels and in vitro studies of estradiol production by granulosa cells isolated from PCOS, clearly demonstrate that the granulosa cells of follicle from anovulatory women with PCOS remain steroidogenically active and indeed show evidence of increased aromatase activity when compared with follicles of similar size from ovulatory women with either normal or polycystic ovaries[16-18].

Therefore it has been suggested that, in culture, the removal of an endogenous inhibitor of gonadotropins and growth factor action[19] may explain why, under in vitro conditions, these cells become responsive. In order to clarify this aspect we recently evaluated the effect of steroid-free follicular fluid on steroidal response and cell proliferation of human granulosa luteal cells from polycystic and normal ovaries[20].

Granulosa cells (from both PCOS and control patients) were cultured for 48 hours with or without increasing dilutions of follicular fluid obtained from polycystic and normo-ovulating patients. Our results are summarized in figure 1 and 2; they show that both follicular fluids were able to elicit aromatase activity as well as thymidine incorporation, an index of cell proliferation; however granulosa cells from polycystic patients, when incubated with follicular fluid from the same woman, showed a lower increase of aromatase activity with respect to cells incubated with follicular fluid from control subjects. Furthermore the proliferation rate was increased by incubation with either follicular fluid, but the increase was less with the fluid from PCOS subjects compared to that from control women. These data indicate that follicular fluid from polycystic ovaries plays an important role in steroidal response and an even more important role in the regulation of granulosa cells proliferation; this effect may be ascribed to the cumulative effect of several non steroidal compounds contained in the follicular fluid.

It is so conceivable that the pathogenesis of anovulation in PCOS could be ascribed to the effect of an altered message in the cooperation between the granulosa cells and the follicular fluid by preferentially maintaining estradiol synthesis rather than proliferation rate, and lowering the capacity for adequate spontaneous luteinization. These hypotheses seem to be confirmed by our recent paper[21] in which we evaluated the effect of atamestane (a competitive inhibitors of P-450 aromatase) on granulosa luteal cells from polycystic and normal ovaries, showing that the atamestane induced inhibition of basal aromatase activity is markedly more pronounced in granulosa cells from normal ovary than in granulosa from polycystic ovaries. These findings, coupled with the observation that normal follicular growth, selection and ovulation can be induced in some PCOS by administration of exogenous gonadotropins[22] seem to further confirm that locally active factors, rather than defective granulosa cells, are involved in arrested follicle growth in PCOS patients.

It could be hypothesized the presence of specific FSH receptor inhibitors; indeed several studies reported the presence of specific FSH receptor inhibitors of unknown origin in human serum[23,24] and follicular fluid [25,26]. However

Schipper et al.[27], by analyzing the levels of inhibitors of FSH receptor activation in serum and follicular fluid of normogonadotropic anovulatory patients, with or without PCOS, compared to normal controls, did not find significant differences in the studied groups, thus suggesting that these substances do not play a significant role in the regulation of normal and abnormal follicle development. This last finding seems to be in keeping with the observation of a normal, or even high, ovarian steroidogenic response to gonadotropins in vivo; the intravenous administration of FSH in PCOS women is able to elicit the estradiol production to a level similar to that of normoovulatory women[28].

Another hypothesis in order to explain the disparity between inhibited follicle growth and increased steroidogenesis in PCOS could consist in a premature activation of LH-induced mitotic arrest, a phenomenon which is thought to occur normally at the onset of the midcycle LH surge[29] and seem to be related to an increased level of intracellular cyclic AMP (cAMP)[29].

Insulin and growth factors

PCOS has been associated with insulin resistance and hyperinsulinemia[30]; furthermore several data[18,31] have led to the suggestion that, in PCOS subjects, hyperinsulinemia may be responsible for the increased steroidogenesis seen in vitro in granulosa cell cultures, but, paradoxically, by enhancing the response of granulosa cells to LH, may also lead to anovulation. Willis and coworkers[31] proposed that hyperinsulinemia, by increasing the response of granulosa cells to LH, amplifies the effects of LH levels that may already be elevated in these women. Thus, the effect of LH on the maturing follicle is similar to that which, in the normal cycle, is exerted only at the onset of the LH surge. This would be expected to lead to terminal differentiation of granulosa cells, resulting in premature arrest of follicular growth and, hence, failure of ovulation.

The mechanisms of insulin enhanced LH responsiveness remain however to be elucidated; insulin might increase LH receptor number, the affinity of LH for its receptor, or postreceptor responsiveness. Investigations in the porcine system have found that insulin increases LH receptor number and not receptor affinity[32]. The question arises, however, how can the ovary retain its sensitivity to insulin, while traditional insulin sensitive organs, such as liver, fat and muscle, are insulin resistant?

There is a striking similarity between the insulin receptor and type-I Insulin-like Growth Factor (IGF-I) receptor, and it has been postulated that insulin action in the ovary in insulin resistant states may occur via the IGF-I receptor[33,34]. Alternatively insulin could act via a hybrid insulin/IGF-I receptor or via the insulin receptor which may be differentially regulated in the ovary[33].

Human theca-interstizial cells have insulin[35] as well as IGF-I receptors[36]; furthermore Poretsky and colleagues[37] have shown that chronic hyperinsulinemia in female rats upregulated ovarian IGF-I receptors.

In this concern, another issue to be adressed is represented by the IGF system; infact IGF-I is able to stimulate aromatase production by PCOS granulosa cells in culture[18]. Furthermore IGF-I has been shown in rats not only to potentiate FSH action in stimulating essential parameters of granulosa cell function[38], but also to increase the number of ovarian LH receptors[39] and to potentiate the ability of LH to stimulate interstitial/theca cell androgen production[40].

Serum IGF-I concentrations in women with PCOS seem to be within the normal range of those in ovulatory and anovulatory non-PCOS women[41]; also the follicular fluid content of IGF-I seems to be normal in this syndrome[42]. These data do not seem to support a main role of IGF-I as a paracrine factor in the pathogenesis of anovulation in PCOS. On the other hand IGF-I is usually bound to its specific carrier protein, the IGF-Binding Protein-1 (IGF-BP1); this protein is synthesized in the liver, secretory endometrial cells[43] and by granulosa cells[44] and may be involved in transferring IGF-I within the extracellular space[45]. Many studies have demonstrated that serum concentrations of IGF-BP1 are significantly decreased in PCOS and are inversely proportional to serum insulin levels[41,46,47], thus suggesting a main role of insulin in regulating the binding protein concentrations.

Low concentrations of IGF-BP1 in the presence of normal concentration of IGF-I insinuate that, in women with PCOS, levels of free IGF-I are increased; the increase in local IGF-I activity could theoretically contribute to ovarian hyperandrogenism of PCOS. Similarly, increased feed-back activity of IGF-I at the hypothalamic or pituitary level[48] could be related to anovulation. However Cataldo and Giudice[49,50], by examining the profile of IGF-BPs in follicular fluid from atretic and estrogenic follicles from PCOS and normally cycling women, found that IGF-BP2 and IGF-BP4 in follicular fluid from atretic follicles were increased several fold, compared to healthy estrogenic follicles, whereas IGF-BP1 was undetectable.

In view of the abundant IGF-BP2, IGF-BP4 and IGF-BP5 gene expression in PCOS atretic follicle granulosa, theca and stroma[51], it is likely that these IGF-BPs are directly secreted into the follicular fluid of the PCOS follicle. On the light of these considerations it could be so alternatively hypothesized that the increased intrafollicular binding proteins may inhibit IGF action at the follicular level, in particular the FSH potentiation of granulosa cell function, impairing follicular development and dominant follicle selection[33].

Another factor which should be discussed in the pathogenesis of anovulation is represented by the plasminogen activator system; components of this system have been found in the follicular fluid[52] and granulosa cells of human ovaries[53], and plasmin has been shown to weaken the follicular wall in vitro[54]. It also activates the conversion of procollagenase to collagenase, which is required for the breakdown of type IV collagen present in the basement membrane around the grafian follicles at ovulation[55]. Furthermore a positive relation between the plasminogen activator inhibitor 1 (PAI-1), the main regulator of the plasminogen activator system, and insulin resistance, is well established[56].

It could be so hypothesized that in PCOS an insulin related over-production of PAI-1 leads to distorsion in the intraovarian plasminogen-plasmin pathway and anovulation. The first study concerning this issue was reported by Dahlgren and coworkers in 1994[57]; the authors showed that PAI-1 levels were about the same in 28 PCOS patients compared to 56 weight-matched controls. In another study Andersen et al.[58] reported high PAI-1 levels in nine obese patients with polycystic ovaries, and showed a reduction of these levels after dietary intervention. Two further studies seem to confirm the presence of higher PAI-1 levels in PCOS women when compared to normo-ovulatory patients[59,60], thus suggesting the hypothesis that the plasminogen-plasmin pathway might play a significant role in the pathogenesis of anovulation in PCOS.

Not only stimulating growth factors, but also inhibitory growth factors, could be involved in determining anovulatory cycles in PCOS (Table 1). The action of inhibitory growth factors is interesting, particularly epidermal growth factor (EGF), which has been shown to inhibit FSH-stimulated estradiol production by rat granulosa cells[61]. Therefore EGF has been measured in human follicular fluid, aspirated from normal infertile women with regular ovulatory cycles and PCOS patients[62]; the intrafollicular EGF concentrations resulted higher in PCOS group and were inversely related to follicular fluid volume, thus suggesting an important additive role of EGF in the pathogenesis of anovulation in PCOS.

TABLE 1 - *Paracrine modulators of ovarian function.*

Stimulatory action:	– Estrogens
	– Androgens
	– Insulin
	– IGF–I
Inhibitory action:	– TGF
	– TGFß
	– EGF

Transforming growth factor alfa (TGFα) is another potent inhibitor of aromatization in cultured granulosa cells[63]; furthermore it is able to inhibit follicular growth[63]. However Mason and coworkers[64] did not find differences in the intrafollicular levels of TGFα between follicles from normal ovaries and PCOS ones. Also the follicular fluid levels of TGFß2 levels did not differ between anovulatory PCOS and normally cycling women[65].

Metabolic Derangements

In recent years the metabolic implications of polycystic ovary syndrome have received a great deal of attention; infact 50% of women with PCOS are obese and a similar percentage of subjects was found to show exaggerated insulin secretion and reduced insulin-stimulated glucose uptake[30]. Furthermore, although about 70% of obese women with PCOS exhibited an exaggerated insulin secretion, this feature is also represented in 20-40% of lean subjects[66].

The presence of obesity and/or insulin resistance has profound clinical implications in terms of morbidity due to diabetes mellitus, dyslipidemia, hypertension and cardiovascular disease. On the other hand obesity and hyperinsulinemia could constitute two main factors in the developing of chronic anovulation; in the previous section we discussed some potential mechanisms by which hyperinsulinemia could interfere with follicular development at the ovarian level.

The relationship between insulin sensitivity and menstrual patterns in PCOS have been well documented by Kiddy and coworkers[67], who showed a reduced insulin sensitivity in a group of oligomenorrheic PCOS women as compared either to controls or PCOS with regular cycles. In keeping with these data are those by Velazquez et al.[68,69], who showed that metformin therapy was able to reduce insulin resistance while improving menstrual cyclicity in 96% of PCOS patients.

The mechanisms by which insulin could play a role in the pathogenesis of anovulation in PCOS (other than those at the ovarian level) might include an involvement of insulin on gonadotropin levels. Indeed many[68,70,71], but not all[72], studies using insulin-lowering drugs (like as troglitazone and metformin) have shown reduced LH levels in conjunction with suppression of insulin levels in PCOS women, thus suggesting an enhancing influence of insulin on LH secretion. By contrast other investigators[73] showed that obesity in PCOS is associated with an attenuation of LH pulse amplitude and LH response to GnRH, not accounted for obesity *per se*, but also for insulin resistance, thus suggesting a blunting effect of hyperinsulinemia and reduced insulin sensitivity on LH levels in PCOS[74].

In order to clarify the insulin/LH relationship in PCOS we recently analyzed the LH response to GnRH bolus in 110 PCOS patients divided in four groups according to their body mass index and insulin secretion (lean-normoinsulinemic, lean-hyperinsulinemic, obese-normoinsulinemic, obese-hyperinsulinemic)[75]; in our series the hyperinsulinemic groups showed an increased LH response to GnRH stimulus when compared to normoinsulinemic counterparts, even if the difference was significant only within lean subjects.

On the basis of these findings we hypothesized a different impact of hyperinsulinemia in lean and obese PCOS patients; infact in the last ones the main cause of hyperinsulinemia could be represented by reduced peripheral insulin sensitivity, hypothetically present also at the pituitary level. By contrast in lean hyperinsulinemic PCOS patients, who were characterized by an exaggerated insulin response to glucose load without the presence of insulin resistance[76],

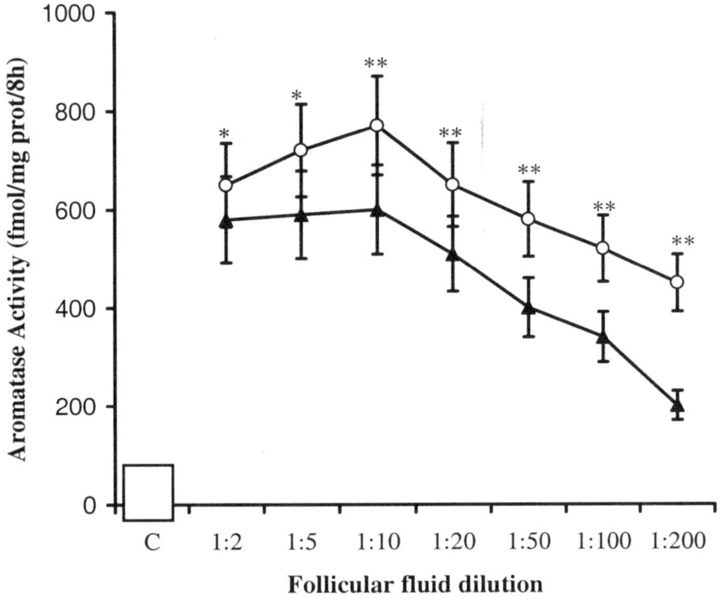

FIGURE 1 - *Aromatase activity of granulosa cells from PCOS patients when treated with follicular fluid from PCOS (▲———▲) or controls (○—— ○) women. Data are expressed as mean ± SEM. Significance: *p<0.05; ** p<0.01 between groups. Modified from reference 20 with permission.*

the increased circulating insulin levels could, directly or indirectly, act by sensitizing gonadotroph cells. This seems to be confirmed by the fact that, in our series, within hyperinsulinemic subjects the obese group showed slightly lower, but not significantly, LH response to GnRH in respect to lean one, in spite of greater secretory response of insulin by ß-cells.

Obesity *per se* is a main cause of insulin resistance; it is so very difficult to distinguish the differential impact of obesity and reduced peripheral insulin sensitivity on the menstrual cycle regulation of PCOS. Indeed it is likely that the first therapeutical approach considered in obese PCOS patients, in order to obtain a restored menstrual cyclicity, should be a dietary regimen; weight loss is invariably associated with an improvement of insulin sensitivity and a reduction in circulating plasma insulin concentrations in PCOS women[58,77].

Since 1982 Bates and Whitworth (78) have described 10 pregnancies in 13 patients with PCOs who lost >15% of their body weight by dietary restriction.

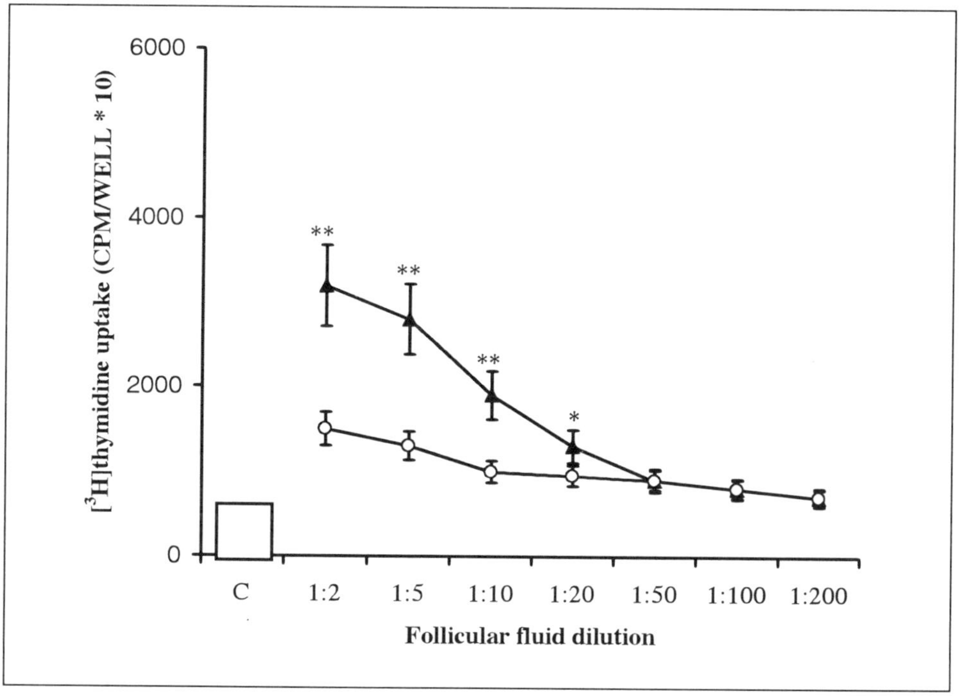

FIGURE 2 - *Cell proliferation (expressed as [^{3}H]thymidine uptake) in granulosa cell cultures from PCOS patients when treated with follicular fluid from PCOS (▲——▲) or controls (○——○) women. Data are expressed as mean ± SEM. Significance: *p<0.05; ** p<0.01 between groups. Modified from reference 20 with permission.*

TABLE 2 - *Possible pathogenetic factors of anovulation in polycystic ovary syndrome.*

– Deficiency of FSH
– Increase of LH
– Increase of insulin
– Obesity
– Increase of androgens
– Increase (or decrease) of growth factors
– Increase of PAI–1

Moreover it is not necessary for a subject to attain her ideal body weight for clinical improvement to be made; with only moderate weight loss (at least 5%) the menstrual function may be restored. Kiddy and coworkers[79] recently reported an analysis of 24 obese PCOS women who underwent a low-calorie/ low-fat diet for 7 months; among the group of 13 patients who loss >5% of their starting weight, 82% of women showed an improvement in ovarian function and five of them (38%) became pregnant.

It could be hypothesized that a main mechanism by which obesity could influence the ovarian function is mediated by an involvement on LH regulation, which in turn could be mediated by insulin. However Guzick et al.[80], by analyzing the effects of weight loss in obese hyperandrogenic, anovulatory women, did not find changes in LH concentrations, pulse frequency or pulse amplitude after dietary intervention, thus suggesting that weight loss do not influence the hypothalamic or pituitary regulation of LH secretion.

Conclusions

Anovulation in PCOS is characterized by arrested growth of antral follicles at the 5-10 mm. stage. A relative lack of FSH may lead to perpetuation of anovulatory state, but is unlikely, by itself, to be a measure cause of it. Despite arrested growth, granulosa cells from anovulatory women with PCOS hypersecrete estradiol, thus leading to the hypothesis that one or more paracrine factors present in the follicular fluid may interfere with the follicular development. A summary of the possible pathogenetic factors of anovulation is reported in Table 2.

The metabolic derangements of the syndrome may influence the ovarian function, as stated by the restored ovarian cyclicity after dietary regimens and/ or insulin lowering drugs.

In conclusion it could be considered that the mechanisms leading to anovulation in PCOS are very complex in nature and that the metabolic status could constitute a main factor in determining such dysfunction.

References

1. Adams J., Polson D.W., Franks S.: Prevalence of polycystic ovaries in women with anovulation and idiopathic hirsutism. *Br. Med. J.*, 293:355-359, 1986.
2. Hull M.G.: Epidemiology of infertility and polycystic ovarian disease: endocrinological and demographic studies. *Gynecol. Endocrinol.*, 2:235-245, 1987.
3. Franks S., Mason H.D., Polson D.W., Winston R.M.L., Margara R., Reed M.J.: Mechanism and management of ovulatory failure in women with polycystic ovary syndrome. *Hum. Reprod.*, 3:351-354, 1988.
4. Willis D., Mason H., Gilling-Smith C., Franks S.: Modulation by insulin of follicle-stimulating hormone and luteinizing hormone actions in human granulosa cells of normal and polycystic ovaries. *J. Clin. Endocrinol. Metab.*, 81:302-309, 1996.
5. Marshall J.C., Griffin M.L.: The role of changing pulse frequency in the regulation of ovulation. *Hum. Reprod.*, 8(Suppl. 2):57-61, 1993.
6. Kazer R.R., Kessel B., Yen S.S.C.: LH pulse frequency in women with PCOS. *J. Clin. Endocrinol. Metab.*, 65:223-226, 1987.
7. Waldstreicher J., Santoro N.F., Hall J.E., Filicori M., Crowley W.F.: Hyperfunction of the hypothalamic pituitary axis in women with PCOS. *J. Clin. Endocrinol. Metab.*, 66:165-172, 1988.
8. Rossmanith W.G., Yen S.S.C.: Sleep associated decrease in luteinizing hormone pulse frequency during the early follicular phase of the menstrual cycle: evidence for an opioidergic mechanism. *J. Clin. Endocrinol. Metab.*, 65:715-718, 1987.
9. Zumoff B., Freemann R., Coupey S., Saenger P., Markowitz M., Kreanin K.: A chronobiologic abnormality in luteinizing hormone secretion in teenage girls with the polycystic ovary syndrome. *N. Engl. J. Med.*, 309:1206-1209, 1983.
10. McNatty K.P., Sawers R.S., McNeilly A.S.: A possible role for prolactin in control of steroid secretion by the human Graafian follicle. *Nature*, 250:653-658, 1984.
11. Soules M.R., Steiner R.A., Clifton D.K., Cohen N.L., Aksel S., Bremner W.J.: Progesterone modulation of pulsatile luteinizing hormone secretion in normal women. *J. Clin. Endocrinol. Metab.*, 58:378-383, 1984.
12. Moenter S.M., Caraty A., Locatelli A., Karsch F.J.: Pattern of GnRH secretion leading up to ovulation in the ewe: existence of a preovulatory GnRH surge. *Endocrinology*, 129:1175-1182, 1991.
13. Dunaif A.: Do androgens directly regulate gonadotropin secretion in polycystic ovary syndrome? *J. Clin. Endocrinol. Metab.*, 63:215-221, 1986.

14. Chang R.I., Mandel F.P., Liu J.K.H., Judd H.L.: Enhanced disparity of gonadotropin secretion by estrone in women with polycystic ovarian disease. *J. Clin. Endocrinol. Metab.*, 54:490-494, 1982.
15. Schaison G.: Pathophysiology of anovulation. *Hum. Reprod.*, 3:525-530, 1988.
16. Erickson G.F., Magoffin D.A., Garzo G.V., Cheung A.P., Chang R.J.: Granulosa cells of polycystic ovaries: are they normal or abnormal? *Hum. Reprod.*, 7:293-299, 1992.
17. Mason H.D., Willis D.S., Beard R.W., Winston R.M.L., Margara R., Franks S.: Estradiol production by granulosa cells of normal and polycystic ovaries: relationship to menstrual cycle hystory and to concentrations of sex steroids in follicular fluid. *J. Clin. Endocrinol. Metab.*, 79:1355-1360, 1994.
18. Andreani C.L., Pierro E., Lanzone A., Lazzarin N., Capitanio G., Giannini P., Mancuso S.: Effects of gonadotropins, insulin and IGF-I on granulosa luteal cells from polycystic ovaries. *Mol. Cell. Endocrinol.*, 106:91-97, 1994.
19. Franks S., Mason H.D.: Polycystic ovary syndrome interaction of follicle stimulating hormone and polypeptide growth factors in estradiol production by human granulosa cells. *J. Steroid Biochem. Mol. Biol.*, 40:405-409, 1991.
20. Andreani C.L., Pierro E., Lazzarin N., Lanzone A., Caruso A., Mancuso S.: Effect of follicular fluid on granulosa luteal cells from polycystic ovaries. *Hum. Reprod.*, 11:2107-2113, 1996.
21. Pierro E., Andreani C.L., Lazzarin N., Cento R., Lanzone A., Caruso A., Mancuso S.: Further evidence of increased aromatase activity in granulosa luteal cells from polycystic ovary. *Hum. Reprod.*, 12:1890-1896, 1997.
22. Fulghesu A.M., Villa P., Pavone V., Guido M., Apa R., Caruso A., Lanzone A., Rossodivita A., Mancuso S.: The impact of insulin secretion on the ovarian response to exogenous gonadotropins in polycystic ovary syndrome. *J. Clin. Endocrinol. Metab.*, 82:644-8, 1997.
23. Reichert Jr L.E., Sanzo M.A., Darga N.S.: Studies on a low molecular weight follicle-stimulating hormone binding inhibitor from human serum. *J. Clin. Endocrinol. Metab.*, 49:866-872, 1979.
24. Sanzo M.A., Reichert Jr L.E.: Gonadotropin receptor binding regulators in serum: characterization and separation of follitropin binding inhibitor and lutropin binding stimulator. *J. Biol. Chem.*, 257:6033-6040, 1982.
25. Fletcher P.W., Dias J.A., Sanzo A., Reichert Jr L.E.: Inhibition of FSH action on granulosa cells by low molecular weight components of follicular fluid. *Mol. Cell Endocrinol.*, 25:303-315, 1982.
26. Lee D.W., Grasso R., Dattatreyamurty B., Deziec M.R., Reichert Jr L.E.: Purification of a high molecular weight follicle-stimulating hormone re-

ceptor-binding inhibitor from human follicular fluid. *J. Clin. Endocrinol. Metab.*, 77:163-168, 1993.

27. Schipper I., Rommerts F.F.G., Ten Hagen P.M., Fauser B.C.J.M.: Low levels of follicle-stimulating hormone receptor-activation inhibitors in serum and follicular fluid from normal controls and anovulatory patients with or without polycystic ovary syndrome. *J. Clin. Endocrinol. Metab.*, 82:1325-1331, 1997.
28. Caruso A., Fortini A., Fulghesu A.M., Pistilli E., Cucinelli F., Lanzone A., Mancuso S.: Ovarian sensitivity to follicle-stimulating hormone during the follicular phase of the human menstrual cycle and in patients with polycystic ovarian syndrome. *Fertil. Steril.*, 59:115-120, 1993.
29. Hillier S.G.: Current concepts of the roles of follicle stimulating hormone and luteinizing hormone in folliculogenesis. *Hum. Reprod.*, 9:188-191, 1994.
30. Ciampelli M., Lanzone A.: Insulin and polycystic ovary syndrome: a new look at an old subject. *Gynecol. Endocrinol.*, (in press), 1998.
31. Willis D., Mason H., Gilling-Smith C., Franks S.: Modulation by insulin of follicle-stimulating hormone and luteinizing hormone action in human granulosa cells of normal and polycystic ovaries. *J. Clin. Endocrinol. Metab.*, 81:302-309, 1996.
32. May J.V., McCarthy Jr K., Reichert Jr L.E., Schomberg D.W.: Follicle-stimulating hormone-mediated induction of functional luteinizing hormone / human chorionic gonadotropin receptors during monolayer culture of porcine granulosa cells. *Endocrinology*, 111:614-624, 1980.
33. Giudice L.C.: Insulin-like growth factors and ovarian follicular development. *Endocr. Rev.*, 13:641-669, 1992.
34. Barbieri Rl., Smith S., Ryan K.J.: The role of hyperinsulinism in the pathogenesis of ovarian hyperandrogenism. *Fertil. Steril.*, 50:197-205, 1988.
35. Poretsky L., Grigorescu F., Flier J.S.: *Insulin but not IGF-I receptors are widely distributed in normal human ovary.* Program of the 67th Annual Meeting of the Endocrine Society, Baltimore MD, Abstract 814, 1985.
36. Poretsky L., Bhargava G., Levitan E.: Type I insulin-like growth factors receptors in human ovarian stroma. *Horm. Res.*, 33:22-7, 1990.
37. Poretsky L., Glover B., Laumas V., Kalin M., Dunaif A.: The effects of experimental hyperinsulinemia on steroid secretion, ovarian [^{125}I] insulin binding and ovarian [^{125}I] insulin-like growth factor-I binding in the rat. *Endocrinology*, 122:581-588, 1988.
38. Adashi E.Y., Resnick C.E., D'Ercole A.J., Svodoba M.E., Van Ben J.J.: Insulin-like growth factors as intraovarian regulators of granulosa cell growth and function. *Endocr. Rev.*, 6:400-420, 1985.
39. Cara J.F., Rosenfield R.L.: Somatomedin-C/insulin like growth factor-I

(IGF-I) enhances LH binding to rat ovarian theca-interstitial cells. *Clin. Res.*, 36:901A-910A, 1988.

40. Cara J.F., Rosenfield R.L.: Insulin-like growth factor-I and insulin potentiate luteinizing hormone-induced androgen synthesis by rat ovarian thecal-interstitial cells. *Endocrinology*, 123:733-739, 1988.
41. Homburg R., Pariente C., Lunenfel B., Jacobs H.S.: The role of insulin-like growth factor-1 (IGF-1) and IGF binding protein 1 (IGFBP-1) in the pathogenesis of polycystic ovary syndrome. *Hum. Reprod.*, 7:1379-1383, 1992.
42. Eden J.A., Jones J., Carter G.D., Alaghband-Zadem J.: Follicular fluid concentrations of insulin like growth factor 1, epidermal growth factor, transforming growth factor-alpha and sex steroids in volume matched normal and polycystic human follicles. *Clin. Endocrinol.*, (Oxf). 32:395-405, 1990.
43. Julkunen M., Koistinen R., Aalto-Setala K., Seppala M., Janne D., Kontuia K.: Primary structure of human insulin-like growth-factor binding protein/ placental protein 12 and tissue specific expression of its mRNA. *FEBS Lett.*, 236:295-301, 1988.
44. Koistinen R., Unterman T.G., Glick R.P., Tiitinen A., Kontula K., Seppala M.: Human granulosa cells contain insulin-like growth factor binding protein-1 (IGFBP-1) mRNA. *Clin. Endocrinol.* (Oxf)., 32:635-640, 1990.
45. Geisthovel F., Moretti-Rojas I., Rojas F.J., Asch R.H.: Insulin-like growth factors and theca-granulosa-cell function. *Hum. Reprod.*, 5:785-799, 1990.
46. Conway G.S., Jacobs H.S., Holly J.M.P., Wass J.A.H.: Effects of luteinizing hormone, insulin, insulin-like growth factor-binding protein in patients with polycystic ovary syndrome. *Hum Reprod.*, 4:136-9, 1989.
47. Suikkari AM, Ruutianen K, Erkkola R, Seppala M. Low levels of low molecular weight insulin-like growth factor-binding protein in patients with polycystic ovary syndrome. *Hum. Reprod.*, 4:136-139, 1989.
48. Ceda G.P., Davis R.G., Rosenfield R.G., Hoffman A.R.: The growth hormone (GH)-releasing hormone (GHRH)-GH-somatomedin axis: evidence for rapid inhibition of GHRH-elicited GH release by insulin-like growth factors 1 and 2. *Endocrinology*, 120:1658-1662, 1987.
49. Cataldo N.A., Giudice L.C.: Insulin-like growth factor binding protein profiles in human ovarian follicular fluid correlate with follicular functional status. *J. Clin. Endocrinol. Metab.*, 74:821-826, 1992.
50. Cataldo N.A., Giudice L.C.: Follicular fluid insulin-like growth factor binding protein profiles in polycystic ovary syndrome. *J. Clin. Endocrinol. Metab.*, 74:695-700, 1992.
51. El-Roeiy A., Roberts V.J., Shimasaki S., Ling N., Yen S.S.C.: *Localization, expression of insulin-like growth factor binding protein (IGFBP-1) 1-6 in normal and polycystic ovaries.* Program of the 48th Annual Meeting of The American

Fertility Society, New Orleans, LA, p. S9 (Abstract 0-020), 1992.
52. Andolf E., Casslen B., Jorgensen C., Buchhave P., Lecander I.: Fluid characteristics of benign ovarian cysts: correlation with recurrence after puncture. *Obstet. Gynecol.*, 86:529-535, 1995.
53. Piquette G.N., Crabtree M.E., Imam E.-D., Milki A., Polan L.: Regulation of plasminogen activator inhibitor-1 and -2 messenger ribonucleic acid levels in human cumulus and granulosa-luteal cells. *J. Clin. Endocrinol. Metab.*, 76:518-523, 1993.
54. Beers W.H.: Follicular plasminogen and plasminogen activator and the effect of plasmin on ovarian follicle wall. *Cell*, 6:379-386, 1975.
55. Puistola U., Westerlund A., Kauppila A., Turpeeniemi Hujanen T.: Regulation of 72 Kd type IV collagenase matrix metalloproteinase-II by estradiol and gonadotropin-releasing hormone agonist in human granulosa lutein cells. *Fertil. Steril.*, 64:81-87, 1995.
56. Juhan-Vague C., Roul M.C., Alesi J.P., Ardissone M., Heim M., Vague P.: Increased plasminogen activator inhibitor activity in non-insulin dependent diabetes – relationship with plasma insulin. *Thromb. Haemost.*, 61:370-373, 1989.
57. Dalghren E., Jansen O.P., Johansson S., Lapidus L., Lindstedt G., Tengborn L.: Haemostatic and metabolic variables in women with polycystic ovary syndrome. *Fertil. Steril.*, 61:455-460, 1994.
58. Anderson P., Seljeflo I., Abdelnoor M., Arnesen H., Dale P.O., Lovik A.: Increased insulin sensitivity and fibrinolytic capacity after dietary intervention in obese women with polycystic ovary syndrome. *Metabolism*, 44:611-616, 1995.
59. Sampson M., Kong C., Patel A., Unwin R., Jacobs H.S.: Ambulatory blood pressure profiles and plasminogen activator inhibitor (PAI-I) in lean women with and without the polycystic ovary syndrome. *Clin. Endocrinol.* (Oxf)., 45:623-629, 1996.
60. Atiomo W.U., Bates S.A., Condon J.E., Shaw S., West J.H., Prentice A.G.: The plasminogen activator system in women with polycystic ovary syndrome. *Fertil. Steril.*, 69:236-241, 1998.
61. Hsueh A.J.W., Welsh T.H., Jones P.B.C.: Inhibition of ovarian and testicular steroidogenesis by epidermal growth factor. *Endocrinology*, 108:2002-2004, 1981.
62. Franks S., Neagle G., Leake R., Mason H.D., Harlow C., Winston R., Margara R., Reed M.: Epidermal growth factor (EGF) concentrations in follicular fluid from normal or polycystic ovaries (PCOS). *J. Endocrinol.*, (Suppl) 112:Abstract 120, 1987.
63. Almahbobi G., Nagodavi Thane A., Trounson A.D.: Effects of epidermal

growth factor, transforming growth factor a and androstenedione on follicular growth and aromatization in culture. Mol Hum Reprod Vol. 1, *Hum. Reprod.*, 10:2767-2772, 1995.
64. Mason H.D., Carr L., Leake R., Franks S.: Production of transforming growth factor a by normal and polycystic ovaries. *J. Clin. Endocrinol. Metab.*, 80:2053-2056, 1995.
65. Barreca A., Del Monte P., Ponzani P., Artini P.G., Genazzani A.R., Minuto F.: Intrafollicular insulin-like growth factor II levels in normally ovulating women and in patients with polycystic ovary syndrome. *Fertil. Steril.*, 65:739-745, 1996.
66. Lanzone A., Fulghesu A.M., Andreani C.L., Apa R., Fortini A., Caruso A., Mancuso S.: Insulin secretion in polycystic ovarian disease: effect of ovarian suppression by GnRH agonist. *Hum. Reprod.*, 5:143-149, 1990.
67. Kiddy R.D., Gelding S.V., Willis D., Bithy Ananthan S., Bush A., Johnston D.G., Franks S.: The relationship of insulin insensitivity and menstrual pattern in women with hyperandrogenism and polycystic ovaries. *Clin. Endocrinol.* (Oxf)., 39:351-355, 1993.
68. Velazquez E.M., Mendoza S., Hamer T., Sosa F., Glueck C.J.: Metformin therapy in polycystic ovary syndrome reduces hyperinsulinemia, insulin resistance, hyperandrogenemia and systolic blood pressure, while facilitating normal menses and pregnancy. *Metabolism*, 43:647-654, 1994.
69. Velazquez E.M., Acosta A., Mendoza S.G.: Menstrual ciclicity after metformin therapy in polycystic ovary syndrome. *Obstet. Gynecol.*, 90:392-395, 1997.
70. Nestler J.E., Jakubowicz D.J.: Decreases in ovarian cytochrome P450 c17a activity and serum free testosterone after reduction of insulin secretion in polycystic ovary syndrome. *N. Engl. J. Med.*, 335:617-623, 1996.
71. Dunaif A., Scott D., Finegood D., Quintana B., Whitcomb R.: The insulin-sensitizing agent troglitazone improves metabolic and reproductive abnormalities in the polycystic ovary syndrome. *J. Clin. Endocrinol. Metab.*, 81:3299-3306, 1996.
72. Ehrman D.A., Schneider D.J., Sobel B.E., Cavaghan M., Imperial J., Rosenfeld R.L., Polonsky K.S.: Troglitazone improves defects in insulin action, insulin secretion, ovarian steroidogenesis and fibrinolysis in women with polycystic ovary syndrome. *J. Clin. Endocrinol. Metab.*, 82:2108-2116, 1997.
73. Morales A.J., Laughlin G.A., Butzo W.T., Maheshwari H., Bauman G., Yen S.S.C.: Insulin, somatotropic, and luteinizing hormone axes in lean and obese women with polycystic ovary syndrome: common and distinct features. *J. Clin. Endocrinol. Metab.*, 81:2854-2864, 1996.
74. Arroyo A., Laughlin G.A., Morales A.J., Yen S.S.C.: Inappropriate gonado-

tropin secretion in polycystic ovary syndrome: influence of adiposity. *J. Clin. Endocrinol. Metab.*, 82:3728-3733, 1997.

75. Ciampelli M., Fulghesu A.M., Cucinelli F., Pavone V., Ronsisvalle E., Guido M., Caruso A., Lanzone A.: Impact of insulin and body mass index on metabolic and endocrine variables in polycystic ovary syndrome. *Metabolism,* (in press), 1998.
76. Ciampelli M., Fulghesu A.M., Cucinelli F., Pavone V., Caruso A., Mancuso S., Lanzone A.: Heterogeneity in ß-cell activity, hepatic insulin clearance and peripheral insulin sensitivity in women with polycystic ovary syndrome. *Hum. Reprod.*, 12:1897-1901, 1997.
77. Holte J., Bergh T., Berne C., Wide L., Lithell H.: Restored insulin sensitivity but persistently increased early insulin secretion after weight loss in obese women with polycystic ovary syndrome. *J. Clin. Endocrinol. Metab.*, 80:2586-2593, 1995.
78. Bates G.N., Whitworth N.S.: Effects of body weight reduction on plasma androgens in obese infertile women. *Fertil. Steril.*, 38:406-409, 1982.
79. Kiddy D.S., Hamilton-Fairley D., Bush A., Short F., Anyaoku V., Reed M.J.: Improvement in endocrine and ovarian function during dietary treatment of obese women with polycystic ovary syndrome. *Clin. Endocrinol.* (Oxf), 36:105-111, 1992.
80. Guzick D.S., Wing R., Smith D., Berga S.L., Winters S.J.: Endocrine consequences of weight loss in obese, hyperandrogenic, anovulatory women. *Fertil. Steril.*, 61:598-604, 1994.

The Role of Luteinizing Hormone
in Folliculogenesis
and Ovulation Induction, pp. 135-143
Editor M. Filicori

Effects of Different Menotropin Preparations for Assisted Reproduction in Hypogonadotropic Hypogonadism

U.D. Gordon

Center for Reproductive Medicine, University of Bristol, Bristol (United Kingdom)

Abstract. *Comparison of different menotropin preparations in hypogonadotropic hypogonadal women has been almost exclusively undertaken in ovulation induction studies. These have confirmed that follicular growth can be achieved using follicle stimulating hormone (FSH) alone, however, serum estradiol* (E_2) *concentrations are extremely low when compared to menotropins where FSH/luteinising hormone (LH) content is equivalent. These studies also demonstrate that, using FSH alone, the overall number of dominant follicles is lower and ovulation is compromised in a large percentage of cases while endometrial thickness and luteal phase progesterone levels are reduced.*

Todate, only a single report has compared different menotropins for assisted reproduction in hypogonadotropic hypogonadism patients. Recombinant FSH (rhFSH), human menopausal gonadotropin (hMG) and purified urinary FSH (uFSH) plus oestradiol valerate were compared in a woman with gonadotropin deficiency. The total number of gonadotropin ampoules used was lower in the hMG treatment cycle with a higher number of follicles and oocytes. The fertilisation rate was significantly higher (93%) compared to rhFSH (28%) and uFSH plus oestradiol valerate (27%) treatment.

In vitro embryo developmental potential as studied in gonadotropin releasing hormone (GnRH)-antagonist treated macaques has also shown that the combination of rhFSH and recombinant LH (rhLH) treatment improves embryo viability and cryosurvival compared to rhFSH alone. In addition, while successfully completed pregnancies and livebirths have been reported in hypogonadal women treated with rhFSH and rhLH, no pregnancies todate have been documented with FSH alone.

In summary, for assisted reproduction in hypogonadotropic hypogonadal women, use of a menotropin preparation containing LH or LH-like activity appears to be essential.

Key words. Hypogonadotropic hypogonadism, assisted reproduction, luteinising hormone, follicle stimulating hormone.

Hypogonadotropic hypogonadism is a heterogeneous condition of varying aetiology. It is characterised by reduced hypothalamic or pituitary activity resulting in abnormally low serum FSH and LH levels and negligible oestrogen activity. Comparison of different menotropin preparations in these women has been almost exclusively undertaken in ovulation induction studies[1,2]. Whilst the aim of ovulation induction in hypogonadotropic women is to induce mono-ovulation and conception in vivo, superovulation for assisted reproduction, on the other hand, requires sufficient number of oocytes for successful fertilisation and cleavage. Todate, only a single report has looked at the effect of different menotropin preparations for assisted reproduction[3].

Determining the optimal amount of LH, or the ratio of FSH:LH needed in the stimulating drugs used therapeutically is a problem that dates back to the early days of gonadotropin therapy[4]. Traditionally, ovulation induction methods used equal amounts of FSH and LH (75:75) in the form of hMG and the 75 IU cut-off point was chosen on an empirical basis rather than on the results of dose-finding studies. Recently, purified preparations of urinary-derived gonadotropins have become available which contain predominantly FSH-related activity (uFSH; Metrodin and Metrodin HP).

Work in macaques on GnRH-antagonist treatment[5], as well as ovulation induction studies in hypogonadotropic women comparing uFSH preparations with hMG suggest that follicular growth can be achieved using uFSH preparations alone. However, serum androstenedione and E_2 concentrations are extremely low. A randomised cross-over study in ten women with complete gonadotropin deficiency showed reduced serum E_2 concentrations with uFSH treatment, with no change in plasma androstenedione levels[1]. Shoham et al.[2], compared hMG treatment with uFSH in subsequent cycles in nine patients with isolated hypogonadotropic hypogonadism and found that the latter treatment required significantly more ampoules of gonadotropin with a reduction in the number of leading follicles, serum E_2 concentrations and endometrial thickness. The above studies also showed that follicles stimulated in the presence of FSH alone did not consistently rupture after human chorionic gonadotropin (hCG) administration. In contrast, studies in women undergoing in vitro fertilisation (IVF) treatment with GnRH-analogues (GnRH-a) and uFSH, showed ovarian responses similar to that of hMG[6-8]. However, it is recognised that in normal women, treatment with GnRH-a does not usually result in total elimination of LH and circulating levels of LH can be measured for a considerable duration[9,10]. In addition, urinary FSH preparations contain varying degrees of LH contamination[11], and therefore, these studies do not conclusively negate the role for LH.

With the advent of recombinant DNA technology and the availability of recombinant gonadotropins[12], it is now possible to revisit and understand the precise roles of FSH and LH in follicular growth and development. The pharmacokinetic and pharmacodynamic properties of recombinant gonadotropins have been studied in detail[13,14] and rhFSH, devoid of LH activity, has been shown to have in-vitro and in-vivo biological characteristics identical to those of native FSH[15,16]. Studies using rhFSH in hypogonadotropic hypogonadal women have conclusively demonstrated that the two-cell two-gonadotropin concept is applicable to the human model.

Schoot et al.[17] first demonstrated that rhFSH alone can induce follicular growth to the pre-ovulatory stage in a woman with isolated gonadotropin deficiency. However, serum E_2 and follicular fluid E_2 and androstenedione levels were extremely low suggesting that LH is needed for androstenedione biosynthesis as substrate for aromatase activity. Similar findings were subsequently reported in two[18] and seven[19] hypogonadotropic women. The efficacy of rhLH for supporting rhFSH-induced follicular development was investigated in a recent dose-finding study[20]. Recombinant LH was found to promote the ovarian sensitivity to a fixed dose of FSH in terms of follicular development and E_2 secretion. A daily dose of 75 IU rhLH was effective in the majority of hypogonadotropic hypogonadal women in achieving optimal follicular development (defined as 1 follicle 17 mm, 400 pmol/L, midluteal phase progesterone 25 nmol/L), maximal endometrial growth and successful luteinisation when exposed to hCG. Clinical pregnancy rates comparable to that of hMG[21] or pulsatile administration of GnRH[22] were achieved.

A number of IVF studies have compared rhFSH preparations with uFSH[23-27], or hMG[28,29]. However, todate, there is only a single published report comparing different menotropins for assisted reproduction in hypogonadotropic hypogonadism patients[3]. Recombinant FSH, hMG and uFSH plus oestradiol valerate were compared in three IVF cycles in a woman with isolated congenital gonadotropin deficiency. The total number of gonadotropin ampoules used was lower in the hMG treatment cycle with a higher number of follicles and oocytes (Table 1). The fertilisation rate was significantly higher (93%) compared to rhFSH (28%) and uFSH plus oestradiol valerate (27%) treatment. Thirteen embryos resulted from the hMG cycle allowing for the fresh transfer of 3 embryos and two further frozen embryo transfer cycles, while 2 and 3 embryos were obtained and replaced with the rhFSH and uFSH treatment cycles respectively. None of the cycles resulted in a pregnancy. Normal pattern of E_2 and inhibin secretion was seen with the hMG treatment cycle while the rhFSH cycle showed a rather small rise in E_2 concentrations and an atypical inhibin pattern. In the uFSH cycle, oestradiol valerate supple-

TABLE 1 - *Ovarian response and oocyte fertilisation outcome to different menotropin preparations in a woman with hypogonadotropic hypogonadism* (Courtesy[3]).

	rhFSH	*hMG*	*uFSH + oestradiol valerate*
No. of ampoules	60	48	56
Duration of stimulation	15	14	15
E_2 day of hCG (pg/ml)	228	5073	257
No. of follicles ≥ 14mm on day of hCG	10	22	15
No. of oocytes	7	14	11
No. of fertilised oocytes (%)	2 (28)	13 (93)	3 (27)

rhFSH = recombinant follicle stimulating hormone, hMG = human menopausal gonadotropin, uFSH = highly purified urinary FSH, hCG = human chorionic gonadotropin.

mentation restored the normal pattern of inhibin seen in the hMG cycle. While both inhibin and E_2 are secreted by the granulosa cells and are indicators of follicular growth, inhibin is considered to be the more direct index of follicular maturation[30]. Luteal plasma progesterone concentrations were much higher in the hMG treatment cycle.

The markedly different fertilisation rates in the above study show that despite normal follicular development, oocyte developmental potential is compromised in an LH depleted environment. Decreased fertilisation rates using uFSH/rhFSH have also been reported in GnRH-a suppressed IVF patients in comparison to hMG treatment[31-34].

Balasch's study[3] does not comment on the cleavage rates or developmental potential of the embryos. However, in vitro embryo developmental potential as studied in GnRH- antagonist treated macaques has shown that the combination of rhFSH and rhLH treatment improves embryo viability and cryosurvival compared to rhFSH alone[35]. Results from IVF studies in normogonadotropic women vary. Whilst some report better cleavage rates[32] and more transferable embryos[31] with hMG treatment compared to uFSH, others show no effect on cryosurvival[36] and blastocyst formation[34]. In addition, while successfully completed pregnancies and livebirths have been reported in hypogonadal women treated with rhFSH and rhLH[37,38], no pregnancies todate have been documented with FSH alone.

In summary, data available comparing different menotropins for assisted reproduction in hypogonadotropic hypogonadal females is limited to one published report in humans. This is mainly because of the rarity of the condition which precludes recruitment of a large number of patients. In addition, there is the inherent difficulty in the outcome variables for clinical trials involved in this issue. The only acceptable outcome for such studies, involved in comparison of different gonadotropin preparations, is pregnancy. Unfortunately, to demonstrate that small differences in pregnancy rates are statistically significantly different requires that a prohibitively large number of women be prospectively evaluated.

From the available evidence to date, both experimental and clinical, from human and non-human studies, it appears that LH plays an important role not only in ovarian steroidogenesis but also in the optimal development of the follicle and oocyte. For successful assisted reproduction in hypogonadotropic hypogonadal women, use of a menotropin preparation containing LH or LH-like activity appears to be essential. Dose finding studies are now required to evaluate the optimal dosage of LH required to supplement FSH in superovulation in these women.

References

1. Couzinet B., Lestrat N., Brailly S., Forest M., Schaison G.: Stimulation of ovarian follicular maturation with pure follicle stimulating hormone in women with gonadotropin deficiency. *J. Clin. Endocrinol. Metab.*, 66:552-556, 1988.
2. Shoham Z., Balen A., Patel A., Jacobs H.S.: Results of ovulation induction using human menopausal gonadotropins or purified follicle-stimulating hormone in hypogonadotropic hypogonadism patients. *Fertil. Steril.*, 56: 1048-1053, 1991.
3. Balasch J., Miro F., Burzaco I., Casamitjama R., Scivico S., Ballesca J.L., Puerto B., Vanrell J.A.: The role of luteinising hormone in human follicle development and oocyte fertility: evidence from *in-vitro* fertilisation in a woman with long-standing hypogonadotropic hypogonadism and using recombinant human follicle stimulating hormone. *Hum. Reprod.*, 10(7):1678-1683, 1995.
4. Jacobson A., Marshall J.R.: Ovulatory response rate with human menopausal gonadotropins of varying FSH:LH ratios. *Fertil Steril.*, (20):171-178, 1969.
5. Kenigsberg D., Littman B.A., Williams R.F., Hodgen G.D.: Medical hypophysectomy: II. Variability of ovarian response to gonadotropin therapy. *Fertil. Steril.*, 42:116-126, 1984.
6. Lavy G., Pellicer A., Diamond M.P., de Cherney A.H.: Ovarian stimulation for in vitro fertilisation and embryo transfer, human menopausal gonadotropin versus pure human follicle stimulating hormone: a randomised prospective study. *Fertil. Steril.*, 50(1):74-78, 1988.

7. Bentick B., Shaw R.W., Iffland C.A., Burford G., Bernard A.: A randomised comparative study of purified follicle stimulating hormone and human menopausal gonadotropin after pituitary desensitisation with buserelin for superovulation and in vitro fertilisation. *Fertil Steril.*, 50:79-84, 1988.
8. Hull M.G.R., Armatage R.J., McDermott A.: Use of follicle stimulating hormone alone (urofollitropin) to stimulate the ovaries for assisted conception after pituitary desensitisation. *Fertil. Steril.*, 62:997-1003, 1994.
9. Cedars M.I., Lapolt P., Surrey E., Meldrum D.R., Hamilton F.: Leuprolide acetate lowers circulating bioactive luteinising hormone and testosterone concentrations during ovarian stimulation for oocyte retrieval. *Fertil. Steril.*, 53:627-631, 1990.
10. Parinaud J., Oustry P., Perineau M., Reme J.-M., Monrozies, Pontonnier G.: Randomised trial of three luteinising hormone - releasing hormone analogues used for ovarian stimulation in an in vitro fertilization programme. *Fertil. Steril.*, 57:1265-1268, 1992.
11. Giudice E., Crisci C., Eshkol A., Papoian R.: Composition of commercial gonadotropin preparations extracted from human post-menopausal urine: characterisation of non-gonadotropin proteins. *Hum. Reprod.*, 9:2291-2299, 1994.
12. Keene J.L., Matzuk M.M., Otani T., Fauser B.C., Galway A.B., Hsueh A.J., Boime I.: Expression of biologically active human follitropin in Chinese hamster ovary cells. *J. Biol. Chem.*, 246:4769-4775, 1989.
13. Le Cotonnec J.-Y., Porchet H.C., Beltraimi V., Khan A., Toon S., Rowland M.: Clinical pharmacology of recombinant human follicle stimulating hormone (FSH). I. Comparative pharmacokinetics with urinary human FSH. *Fertil. Steril.*, 61:669-678, 1994.
14. Le Cotonnec J.-Y., Porchet H.C., Beltram V., Khan A., Toon S., Rowland M.: Clinical pharmacology of recombinant human follicle stimulating hormone (FSH). II. Single doses and steady state pharmacokinetics. *Fertil. Steril.*, 61:679-686, 1994.
15. Mannaerts B., de Leeuw R., Geelen J., van Ravestein A., van Wezenbeek P., Schuurs A., Kloosterboer H.: Comparative in vitro and in vivo studies on the biological characteristics of recombinant human follicle stimulating hormone. *Endocrinology*, 129:2623-2630, 1991.
16. Porchet H.C., Le Cotonnec J.-Y., Canali S., Zanolo G.: Pharmaco-kinetics of recombinant human follicle-stimulating hormone after intravenous, intramuscular and subcutanteous administration in monkeys, and comparison with intravenous administration of urinary follicle stimulating hormone. *Drug Metab. Disposition*, 21:144-150, 1993.
17. Schoot D.C., Coelingh Bennink H.J.T., Mannaerts B.M.L.J., Lamberts

S.W.J., Bouchart P., Fauser B.C.J.M.: Human recombinant follicle stimulating hormone induces growth of preovulatory follicles without concomitant increase in androgen and oestrogen biosynthesis in a woman with isolated gonadotropin deficiency. *J. Clin. Endocrinol. Metab.*, 74:1471-1473, 1992.

18. Shoham Z., Mannaerts B., Insler V., Coelingh-Bennick H.: Induction of follicular growth using recombinant human follicle stimulating hormone in two volunteer women with hypogonadotropic hypogonadism. *Fertil. Steril.*, 59:738-742, 1993.
19. Schoot D.C., Harlin J., Shoham Z., Mannaerts B.M.L.J., Lahlou N., Bouchart P., Coelingh Bennink H.J.T., Fauser B.C.J.M.: Recombinant human follicle stimulating hormone and ovarian response in gonadotropin deficient women. *Hum. Reprod.*, 9:1237-1242, 1994.
20. The European Recombinant Human LH Study Group: Recombinant human luteinising hormone (LH) to support recombinant human follicle stimulating hormone (FSH)-induced follicular development in LH- and FSH-deficient anovulatory women: a dose-finding study. *J. Clin. Endocrinol. Metab.*, 83(5):1507-1514, 1998.
21. Martin K.A., Hall J.E., Adams J.M., Crowley Jr. W.F.: Comparison of exogenous gonadotropins and pulsatile gonadotropin-releasing hormone for induction of ovulation in hypogonadotropic amenorrhea. *J. Clin. Endocrinol. Metab.*, 77:125-129, 1993.
22. Filicori M., Flamigni C., Dellai P., Cognigni G., Michelacci L., Arnone R., Sambataro M., Falbo A.: Treatment of anovulation with pulsatile gonadotropin-releasing hormone prognostic factors and clinical results in 600 cycles. *J. Clin. Endocrinol. Metab.*, 79:1215-1220, 1994.
23. Out H.J., Mannaerts B.M., Driessen S.G., Coelingh-Bennink H.J.: A prospective, randomised, assessor-blind, multi-centre study comparing recombinant and urinary follicle-stimulating hormone (Puregon versus Metrodin) in in-vitro fertilisation. *Hum. Reprod.*, 10(10):2534-2540, 1995.
24. Out H.J., Mannaerts B.M., Driessen S.G.: Recombinant follicle-stimulating hormone (r-hFSH) in assisted reproduction: more oocytes, more pregnancies. Results from five comparative studies. *Hum. Reprod. Update,* 2:162-171, 1996.
25. Recombinant Human FSH Study Group: Clinical assessment of recombinant human follicle stimulating hormone in stimulating ovarian follicular development before in vitro fertilisation. *Fertil. Steril.*, 63:77-86, 1995.
26. Loumaye E., Engrand P., Howles C.M., O'Dea L.: Assessment of the role of serum luteinising hormone and oestradiol response to follicle stimulating hormone on in vitro fertilisation outcome. *Fertil Steril.*, 67(5):889-899, 1997.

27. Bergh C., Howles C.M., Borg K., Hamberger L., Josefsson B., Nilsson L., Wikland M.: Recombinant human follicle stimulating hormone (r-hFSH; Gonal-F) versus highly purified urinary FSH (Metrodin HP): results of a randomised comparative study in women undergoing assisted reproductive techniques. *Hum. Reprod.*, 1210):2133-2139, 1997.
28. Duijkers I.J.M., Willemsen W.M.P., Hollanders J.M.G., Hamilton C.J.C.M., Thomas C.M.G., Vemer H.M.: Follicular fluid hormone concentrations after ovarian stimulation using gonadotrophic preparations with different FSH/LH ratios. II. Comparison of hMG and recombinant FSH. In: Duijkers I.J.M (ed), *Gonadotropins: some basic and clinical aspects,* pp. 143-153, 1995.
29. Jansen C.A.M., Van Os H.C.: Puregon with analogues: an oxymoron. *Gynaecol. Endocrinol.*, 10(Suppl. 1):34-43, 1996.
30. Burger H.G.: Clinical utility of inhibin measurements. *J. Clin. Endocrinol. Metab.*, 76:1391-1396, 1993.
31. Westergaard L.G., Erb K., Laursen S., Rasmussen P.E., Rex S.: The effect of human menopausal gonadotropin and highly purified, urine-derived follicle stimulating hormone on the outcome of in vitro fertilisation in down-regulated normogonadotropic women. *Hum Reprod.*, 11(6):1209-1213, 1996.
32. Soderstrom-Antilla V., Tuija F., Hovatta O.: A randomised comparative study of purified follicle stimulating hormone and human menopausal gonadotropin for ovarian hyperstimulation in an oocyte donation programme. *Hum. Reprod.*, 11:1864-1870, 1996.
33. Gordon U.D., Gordon A.C., Bonnar J., Harrison R.F.: Effect of differing doses of LH on oocyte maturation and fertilisation. Abstracts of the 13th Annual Meeting of the ESHRE, *Hum Reprod.*, p. 53, 1997.
34. Fleming R., Lloyd F., Herbert M., Fenwick J., Griffiths T., Murdoch A.: Effects of profound suppression of LH during controlled ovarian stimulation on follicular activity, oocyte and embryo function in cycles stimulated with purified FSH. *Hum. Reprod.*, 13(9):1788-1792, 1998.
35. Weston A.M., Zelinski-Wooten M.B., Stouffer R.L., Wolf D.P.: Developmental potential of embryos produced by in vitro fertilisation from gonadotropin-releasing hormone antagonist treated macaques stimulated with recombinant human follicle stimulating hormone alone or in combination with luteinising hormone. *Hum. Reprod.*, 11(3):608-613, 1996.
36. Rekha P., Mowat L., Jamieson M.E., Yates R.W., Fleming R.: Effect of profound suppression of luteinising hormone during treatment with gonadotropin releasing hormone analogue and purified follicle stimulating hormone upon development of cryopreserved embryos. *Hum Reprod.*,

13(3):696-698, 1998.
37. Hull M.G.R., Corrigan E., Piazzi A., Loumaye E.: Recombinant human luteinising hormone: an effective new gonadotropin preparation. *Lancet,* 344(8918):334-335, 1994.
38. Kousta E., White D.M., Piazzi A., Loumaye E., Franks S.: Successful induction of ovulation and completed pregnancy using recombinant human luteinising hormone and follicle-stimulating hormone in a woman with Kallmann's Syndrome. *Hum. Reprod.*, 11(1):70-71, 1996.

The Role of Luteinizing Hormone
in Folliculogenesis
and Ovulation Induction, pp. 145-153
Editor M. Filicori

Ovulation Induction in Polycystic Ovary Syndrome: Effect of Different Menotropin Preparations in Regular and Low Dose Regimens

R. Homburg

Fertility Unit, Rabin Medical Centre, Hasharon Hospital (Affiliated to Sackler Medical School, Tel Aviv University), Petah Tikva (Israel)

Abstract. *There are several theoretical reasons for believing that FSH preparations, purified urinary FSH (uFSH) and recombinant FSH (recFSH) may improve efficiency and results of treatment of patients with polycystic ovary syndrome (PCOS) compared with hMG. Administration of FSH will hypothetically correct the relative FSH deficency and redress the high LH:FSH ratio, both prevalent and important factors contributing to anovulation in PCOS. In addition, pure FSH, rather than the additional LH in hMG, was thought to to be more likely to reduce the miscarriage rate and increase chances of conception, both influenced by already high LH concentrations. In practice, uFSH, given for ovulation induction in PCOS, whether in a conventional or low dose regimen, has not influenced follicular recruitment and development or ovulation and pregnancy rates when compared with hMG. Both FSH and hMG decrease endogenous LH concentrations, FSH more than hMG, but the exogenous LH in hMG has very little impact on endogenous LH levels in doses used for ovulation induction in PCOS. Not suprisingly then, FSH has not improved pregnancy or miscarriage rates. The mode of administration appears to be much more important than the preparation used. Comparisons of uFSH with recFSH have, on the whole, shown a greater bioactivity of recFSH for which a lower dose and shorter duration of administration was needed. No clinical advantage in pregnancy rates was either expected or obtained with rec FSH in the dose regimens used for ovulation induction in PCOS.*

Key words. Polycystic ovary syndrome, ovulation induction, gonadotropins, recombinant FSH, urinary FSH, human menopausal gonadotropins.

Introduction

Polycystic ovary syndrome (PCOS) is associated with approximately 75% of women who suffer from infertility due to anovulation[1,2]. It is a very heterogeneous syndrome both in its clinical presentation and laboratory manifestations. The majority of women with anovulation associated with PCOS have menstrual irregularities, usually oligomenorrhea or amenorrhea. The main disturbances in this syndrome are:

1. Abnormal morphology of the ovary, detected by a characteristic hyperechogenic enlarged central stroma and >9 small follicles of 2-9mm diameter on transvaginal ultrasound examination of the ovaries[3].
2. Abnormal steroidogenesis, mainly increased ovarian production of androgens.
3. Insulin resistance and hyperinsulinemia, present in the majority of obese women with PCOS but also in 30-40% of women of normal weight with PCOS[4].
4. Abnormal gonadotrophin secretion, most commonly manifested as increased serum LH concentrations in 40% of women with ultrasonically detected PCO's with a consequent rise in the LH:FSH ratio[5].

The treatment of anovulatory infertility associated with PCOS should be progressive. For the obese women (body mass index, BMI > 25) with insulin resistance and hyperinsulinemia, a low calorie diet should be the first approach. A reduction of 5% or more in body weight is often enough to restore menstruation and ovulation or at least, to facilitate ovulation induction[6]. Loss of weight is associated with a reduction of insulin and androgen concentrations and an increase in sex hormone binding hormone concentrations. Obesity per se has a negative influence on both conception and miscarriage rates[7].

The medical treatment of anovulation associated with PCOS, whatever the preparation used, has basically the same aim; to supply FSH stimulation of the follicles which have arrested in their development. This may be done indirectly using anti-estrogens, usually clomiphene citrate (CC), and, infrequently, with pulsatile gonadotrophin-releasing hormone. Clomiphene citrate will induce ovulation in about 80% of these patients but a pregnancy rate of only approximately 35%[8]. It is our policy to regard a 'clomiphene failure' as non-response to clomiphene in a dose of 150mg/day for 5 days or failure to conceive within 6 cycles during which ovulation was successfully induced.

The next step is direct stimulation of the ovaries with a preparation containing FSH. This treatment is relatively very successful in inducing ovulation, presumably by replenishing a relative deficiency in the action of FSH at the level of the follicle in women with PCOS. However, the path to successful induction of ovulation and pregnancy is notoriously precarious in PCOS for several reasons. The polycystic ovary is very much more sensitive to gonadotrophin stimulation than the normal ovary. This is thought to be due to the fact that the polycystic ovary contains a much larger cohort of small viable follicles capable of responding[9]. For this same reason, multiple follicular development is rife and predisposes to a greater incidence of multiple pregnancies and ovarian hyperstimulation syndrome (OHSS). Hypersecretion of LH during the follicular phase, a condition unique to PCOS, has now been well documented as impeding conception and having a detrimental effect on miscarriage rates[10].

The relevant question to be discussed in this chapter is whether the new, purified FSH preparations now on the market, purified urinary FSH (uFSH), highly purified urinary FSH (uFSH-HP) and recombinant FSH (recFSH) devoid of any LH, can improve the efficiency, results and complications of ovulation induction for PCOS compared with hMG. There were several theoretical reasons for believing that this was possible. Administration of pure FSH will, hypothetically, correct the relative FSH deficiency and redress the high LH:FSH ratio, both prevalent and important factors contributing to anovulation and complications of ovulation induction in PCOS. In addition, pure FSH, rather than the additional LH in hMG, were thought to be more likely to reduce the miscarriage rate and chances of conception, both influenced by already high LH concentrations. Similarly, it was hypothesized that the absence of LH in the new preparations could positively influence the rate of OHSS. Following an examination of the available data on differences in the pharmacodynamics, I will review the relevant clinical trials comparing the effects of the different menotrophin preparations used for the induction of ovulation in PCOS.

Pharmacodynamics of Menotropin Administration in PCOS

Several studies have examined and compared the pharmacodynamics involved following a single dose or repeated doses of the various gonadotrophin preparations in women with PCOS.

Anderson et al.[11] performed a randomized trial comparing the pharmacodynamics in the 24h following a single injection of 150 IU of either uFSH or hMG in 10 women with PCOS. Ten normal ovulatory women were similarly randomized to serve as controls. Serum LH decreased significantly by about 27% following uFSH in PCOS but not at all with hMG which increased LH slightly and transiently after 4 hours. Serum FSH levels were only increased significantly by uFSH but not by hMG in women with PCOS. There was a consequent significant decrease in the LH:FSH ratio in response to uFSH resulting in a ratio similar to the baseline of the controls. Serum estradiol responses were higher and earlier with uFSH than with hMG. This pharmacodynamic data is thus supportive of the theoretical advantages of uFSH over hMG in PCOS, at least with respect to gonadotrophin levels.

In order to examine whether the abnormal levels of hormones in PCOS are corrected during treatment with uFSH, Larsen et al.[12] designed a randomized, double-blind crossover study comparing uFSH and hMG in 12 women with PCOS over 30 cycles. They used a conventional, individually adjusted dosage of uFSH or hMG. There was no significant difference in the dosages of uFSH and hMG required to induce ovulation. The elevated baseline values of serum LH were normalized after a few days of stimulation regardless of which type of gonadotrophin was used. The mean serum values of LH were slightly but insignificantly lower when uFSH was used and the LH:FSH ratio was normalized after a few days treatment with both preparations. There were no significant differences between the two preparations regarding increases in serum concentrations of free testosterone, androstendione, dehydroepiandrosterone and estrone. Sex-hormone binding globulin serum concentrations remained stable with again no difference between stimulation with uFSH and hMG. Venturoli et al.[13] obtained very similar results when comparing the hormonal changes while treating the same patients alternately with uFSH and hMG. The findings of Larsen et al regarding the finding of virtually identical concentrations of LH in the circulation during treatment with uFSH or hMG, were confirmed by Sagle et al.[14] in a randomized study using a low-dose protocol.

During induction of ovulation in women with PCOS using low dose, pulsatile uFSH or hMG, Franks et al.[15] found no significant differences in FSH concentrations during the follicular phase. LH concentrations were also similar in the two groups, tending to fall towards the late follicular phase. They concluded that the LH content of hMG had little impact on endogenous LH concentrations at these doses.

However, Polan et al.[16] measured the follicular fluid concentrations of androgens and found that the testosterone/androstendione ratio was higher when hMG was used rather than uFSH. They theorized that this may make a difference and impair oocyte development.

Employing a different strategy, Fulghesu et al.[17] examined the effect of giving uFSH or hMG in PCOS patients pretreated with gonadotrophin-releasing hormone agonist (GnRHa), thereby neutralizing the effect of endogenous LH and FSH secretion. Serum concentrations of LH, both bio and immunoassayed, were significantly higher in hMG induced cycles and, similarly, androstendione and testosterone temporally related to the higher LH concentrations. FSH and estradiol increased to the same extent with uFSH and hMG.

Comparisons involving recFSH, with hMG[18], with uFSH[19,20] or with highly purified uFSH (uFSH-HP)[21] have dealt almost exclusively with clinical efficacy and safety for use in ovulation induction for PCOS rather than pharmacodynamics. They will be reviewed below but the majority of these studies have shown an increased biopotency of recFSH compared with the urinary preparations. Although the reasons for this are not clear, it may be a function of reliance on the Steelman-Poley bioassay used for calibration which has a poor correlation with clinical response in humans. Other reasons proposed for the apparent differences in biopotency are the differences in isoform profile, pharmaceutical fomulation, in the carbohydrate moieties attached to the molecule of recFSH or the lower percentage of oxidized forms of FSH in recFSH[22]. In a compararive study of recFSH and uFSH-HP in women with PCOS, Balasch et al.[21] found a direct correlation between estradiol and inhibin A concentrations on the day of hCG when using recFSH but not uFSH-HP and suggested this as a further possible reason for the better bioactive performance of recFSH.

Clinical Trials

hMG vs uFSH. Clinical comparisons of hMG and uFSH started to appear in 1987 with increasingly larger series up to the present day but without demonstrating any significant clinical difference between the two preparations. One of the first studies[15] employed pulsatile low dose gonadotrophin therapy, either hMG or uFSH, in 9 women over 19 cycles with hMG and 15 women over 51 cycles with uFSH. They found no difference in the mean dose of FSH required to develop an ovulatory follicle or in the percentage of ovulatory or uni-ovulatory cycles. A similar comparison was performed by Venturoli et al.[13] but using a conventional, individually adjusted step-up protocol with i.m. injections in 43 women with PCOS over 52 cycles. There were no differences between the two preparations in ovulation, pregnancy or miscarriage rates. Serum estradiol levels and the number of maturing follicles were significantly greater and mild to moderate OHSS more prevalent with uFSH.

Our own, randomized, study compared uFSH with hMG, with and without pretreatment with GnRH agonist in a four-armed study in 46 patients over 122 cycles using a conventional dose scheme[23]. Whether using GnRH agonist or not, we could detect no difference in the efficacy and responses obtained between stimulation with uFSH or hMG with respect to ovulation, pregnancy and prevalence of OHSS and similarly to dosage and duration of therapy required. We concluded that pure uFSH had no advantages over hMG, the LH content of hMG having no deleterious effect on the ovary.

A randomized, double blind, crossover study comparing uFSH and hMG[12] on 12 patients in alternate cycles showed no difference in the dose required of the two preparations or in the mean increase of ovarian volume. Using a conventional step-up protocol starting with 150IU following GnRH agonist therapy, Fulghesu et al.[17] found no differences in dosage required. Using this regimen the response was multifollicular and the estradiol/number of follicles and estradiol/ovarian volume ratios were greater with hMG than uFSH. They concluded that while clinical results are no different, the LH content of hMG may have a role in the enhancement of steroid production.

Sagle et al[14] performed a comparative, randomized study of low dose hMG and uFSH in 30 women with PCOS over 75 cycles. The rates of ovulation, pregnancy and monofollicular development were almost identical with uFSH or hMG. Their conclusion serves as an excellent summary of the studies quoted here, i.e. low dose uFSH and hMG are equally successful in inducing ovulation suggesting that the success of treatment depends on the low dose of gonadotropin used rather than the presence or absence of LH in the preparation.

hMG vs recFSH. A trial comparing hMG (8 patients, 26 cycles) with recFSH (14 patients, 40 cycles) administered in a classic low dose protocol in women with PCOS who had suffered severe OHSS with previous conventional therapy did not demonstrate any difference in efficacy[18]. No further cases of OHSS were seen with either uFSH or hMG.

uFSH vs recFSH. Two large, randomized, multicentre studies have compared uFSH with recFSH using the classic low dose protocol in women with WHO Group II infertility. The first[19] involved 196 patients, 96 of whom received Gonal-F (Ares Serono, Geneva, Switzerland) given subcutaneously over 225 cycles and 100 who received uFSH i.m. over 233 cycles. Even with these large numbers and statistical power, no significant differences were seen in the efficacy of the two preparations with regard to the number of follicles, monofollicular ovulations and estradiol levels induced. Similarly, there was no difference in ovulation, pregnancy, miscarriage or multiple pregnancy rates between recFSH and uFSH. An equally large study[20] with a similar design using Puregon (NV Organon, Oss, The Netherlands) compared with uFSH again showed similar ovulation and pregnancy rates but claimed a greater bioactivity of recFSH expressed as a significantly lower total dose and shorter treatment period to reach ovulation. In addition, the mean number of follicles of >12mm and estradiol serum levels were significantly higher and serum FSH levels significantly lower in the recFSH group compared to the uFSH group.

uFSH-HP vs recFSH. A very recent study has compared uFSH-HP and recFSH given subcutaneously in a low dose protocol in 20 women with PCOS[21]. They reported that recFSH has a higher in vivo biopotency than highly purified uFSH as judged by follicular development, hormonal levels and amount of FSH required.

Conclusions

The treatment of women with anovulatory infertility associated with PCOS who do not conceive with clomiphene is usually with gonadotropins. The results are no more than satisfactory and the complications of multiple follicular development and consequent OHSS and multiple pregnancies must always be considered. The emergence of purified urinary or pure recombinant FSH preparations do not appear to have had a significant impact on these features of gonadotropin treatment in this special group of patients. The mode of treatment rather than the LH content of the actual preparation used would appear to be a more important consideration.

References

1. Adams J., Polson D.W., Franks S.: Prevalence of polycystic ovaries in women with anovulation and idiopathic hirsutism. *Br. Med. J.*, 293:355-359, 1986.
2. Hull M.G.: Epidemiology of infertility and polycystic ovarian disease: endocrinological and demographic studies. *Gynaecol. Endocrinol.*, 1:235-245, 1987.
3. Adams J., Franks S., Polson D.W., Mason H.D., Abdulwahid N., Tucker M., Morris D.V., Price J., Jacobs H.S.: Multifollocular ovaries: clinical and endocrine features and response to pulsatile gonadotrophin releasing hormone. *Lancet,* ii:1375-78, 1985
4. Dunaif A., Segal K., Futterweit W., Dobrjansky A.: Profound peripheral resistance independent of obesity in polycystic ovary syndrome. *Diabetes,* 38:1165-1174. 1989.
5. Balen A.H., Conway G.S., Kaltsas G., Techatrasak K., Manning P.J., West C., Jacobs H.S.: Polycystic ovary syndrome: the spectrum of the disorder in 1741 patients. *Hum Reprod.*, 10:2107-11, 1995.
6. Kiddy D.S., Hamilton-Fairley D., Bush A., Anyaoku V., Reed M.J., Franks S.:

Improvement in endocrine and ovarian function during dietary treatment of obese women with polycystic ovary syndrome. *Clin. Endocrinol.*, 36: 105-111, 1992.
7. Clark A.M., Thornley B., Tomlinson L., Galletley C., Norman R.J.: Weight loss in obese fertile women results in reproductive outcome for all forms of fertility treatment. *Hum. Reprod.*, 13:1502-1505, 1998.
8. MacGregor A.H., Johnson J.E., Bunde C.A.: Further clinical experience with clomiphene citrate. *Fertil. Steril.*, 19:616-622, 1968.
9. Van der Meer M., Hompes P., de Boer J., Schats R., Schoemaker J.: Cohort size rather than follicle-stimulating hormone threshold levels determines ovarian sensitivity in polycystic ovary syndrome. *J. Clin. Endocrinol. Metab.*, 83:423-426, 1998.
10. Homburg R., Armar N.A., Eshel A., Adams J., Jacobs H.S.: Influence of serum luteinizing hormone concentrations on ovulation, conception and early pregnancy loss in polycystic ovary syndrome. *Br. Med. J.*, 297:1024-1026, 1988.
11. Anderson R.E., Cragun J.M., Chang R.J., Stanczyk F.Z., Lobo R.A.: A pharmacodynamic comparison of human urinary follicle-stimulating hormone and human menopausal gonadotropin in normal women and polycystic ovary syndrome. *Fertil. Steril.*, 52:216-220, 1989.
12. Larsen T., Larsen J.F., Schioler V., Bostofe E., Felding C.: Comparison of urinary human follicle-stimulating hormone and human menopausal gonadotropin for ovarian stimulation in polycystic ovary syndrome. *Fertil. Steril.*, 53:426-431, 1990.
13. Venturoli S., Paradisi R., Fabbri R., Porcu E., Orsini L.F., Flamigni C.: Induction of ovulation in polycystic ovary: Human menopausal gonadotropin or human urinary follicle stimulating hormone? *Int. J. Fertil.*, 32:66-70, 1987.
14. Sagle M., Hamilton-Fairley D., Kiddy D., Franks S.: A comparative, randomized study of low dose human menopausal gonadotropin and follicle stimulating hormone in women with polycystic ovary syndrome. *Fertil. Steril.*, 55:56-60, 1991.
15. Franks S., Polson D.W., Mason H.D.: Pulsatile low dose gonadotrphin therapy in women with polycystic ovaries. In: Wagner T.O.F., Filicori M. (eds). *Episodic Hormone Secretion: From Basic Science to Clinical Application.* TM-Verlag, Hameln, Germany, pp. 243-47, 1987.
16. Polan M.L., Daniele A., Russel J.B., DeCherney A.H.: Ovulation induction with human menopausal gonadotropin compared to human follicle stimulating hormone results in a significant shift in follicular fluid androgen levels without discernible differences in granulosa-luteal cell function. *J.*

Clin. Endocrinol. Metab., 63:1284-1288, 1986.

17. Fulghesu A.M., Lanzone A., Guida C., Nicoletti M.C., Possi P., LeDonne M., Caruso A., Mancuso S.: Ovulation induction with human menopausal gonadotropin versus FSH after pituitary suppression by gonadotropin releasing hormone agonist in polycystic ovary disease. *J. Reprod. Med.*, 37: 834-840, 1992.
18. Aboulghar M.A., Mansour R.T., Serour G.I., Amin Y.A., Sattar M.A., ElAttar E.: Recombinant follicle stimulating hormone in the treatment of patients with history of severe ovarian hyperstimulation syndrome. *Fertil. Steril.*, 66: 757-760, 1996.
19. Ares-Serono: *A phase III, open, randomised, multicentre study to compare the safety and efficacy of recombinant human follicle stimulating hormone (Gonal-F) administered subcutaneously with that of urinary human follicle stimulating hormone (Metrodin) given intramuscularly, to induce ovulation in WHO Group II anovulatory infertile women.* Ares-Serono Internal Report, 1995.
20. Coelingh Bennink H.J.T., Fauser B.C.J.M., Out H.J.: Recombinant follicle stimulating hormone (FSH;Puregon) is more efficient than urinary FSH (Metrodin) in women with clomiphene citrate resistant, normogonadotropic chronic anovulation: a prospective, multicenter, assessor-blind, randomized, clinical trial. *Fertil. Steril.*, 69:19-25, 1998.
21. Balasch J., Fabregues F., Penarrubia J., Montserrat C., Vidal R., Casamitjana R., Manau D., Vanrell J.A.: Follicular development and hormonal levels following highly purified or recombinant follicle stimulating hormone administration in ovulatory women and WHO Group II anovulatory infertile patients. *J. Assist. Reprod. Genet.*, In press. 1998.
22. Out H.J., Mannaerts B., Driessen S., Coelingh Bennink H.: A prospective, randomized, assessor-blind, multicenter study comparing recombinant and urinary follicle stimulating hormone in in-vitro fertilization. *Hum. Reprod.*, 10:2534-2540, 1995.
23. Homburg R., Eshel A., Kilborn J., Adams J., Jacobs H.S.: Combined luteinizing hormone releasing hormone analogue and exogenous gonadotrophins for the treatment of infertility associated with polycystic ovaries. *Hum. Reprod.*, 5:32-35, 1990.

The Role of Luteinizing Hormone
in Folliculogenesis
and Ovulation Induction, pp. 155-164
Editor M. Filicori

Menotropin and GnRH Analog Regimens in Assisted Reproduction

M. Filicori, G.E. Cognigni, R. Pecorari, F. Galletti and L. Parmegiani

Reproductive Endocrinology Center, University of Bologna, Bologna (Italy)

Abstract. *While initial attempts of* in-vitro *fertilization (IVF) procedures were conducted in spontaneous menstrual cycles or using mild ovarian stimulation with clomiphene citrate, current assisted reproduction techniques (ART) include ovarian stimulation with exogenous gonadotropins combined with gonadotropin-releasing hormone (GnRH) analogs. Another critical development that occurred in the last decade is the progressive abandonment of LH-containing menotropins in favor of purified, highly purified, or recombinant FSH. The combination of these LH-deprived gonadotropin preparation and GnRH analogs has resulted in a follicular stimulation virtually devoid of LH activity. Nevertheless, growing evidence suggests that LH plays an important physiologic and clinical role in this setting. Moderate amounts of LH activity appears to optimize ovulation induction, reduce gonadotropin dose requirements, shorten follicular stimulation, and improve overall outcome of ART, possibly also through estrogen-mediated actions on the oocyte. We conclude that LH plays a valuable role in ovulation induction regimens and that, far from being detrimental, LH activity supplementation is a valuable maneuver to optimize ART.*

Key words. LH, FSH, ovulation induction, folliculogenesis.

Early ovulation induction regimens

Ovulation induction is the basic pharmacological procedure needed to achieve multiple folliculogenesis in all assisted reproduction (AR) techniques. While virtually all AR cycles are presently conducted with some form of ovarian stimulation, this was not always the case. The first successful *in vitro* fertilization attempt and most treatment cycles for a while thereafter were conducted in spontaneous menstrual cycles. Nevertheless, realization that availability of a crop of mature oocytes markedly increased chances of success in this therapy prompted most centers to adopt some form of controlled ovarian stimulation (COS). At the outset clomiphene citrate alone or in combination with human menopausal gonadotropins (hMG) was used but eventually exogenous gonadotropins emerged as the sole stimulatory drug for COS.

Clomiphene citrate is an inexpensive and relatively safe drug and its combination with hMG can reduce gonadotropin dose requirements. However, another pharmacological development tilted the balance against the use of clomiphene i.e. the advent of gonadotropin releasing hormone (GnRH) agonists. Soon after the introduction of COS in ART it became evident that in the course of ovulation induction the midcycle LH surge could be unexpectedly triggered by rising ovarian steroid levels; as a result premature ovulation or follicle luteinization could occur and cause cycle cancellations in up to 30% of cases. In order to identify patients on the verge of spontaneous ovulation close monitoring of LH and progesterone (P) plasma levels with multiple daily determination used to be the rule in AR.

Thus, in the mid-1980s GnRH agonist supplementation was tested in ovulation induction[1] and then successfully applied in most cycles. The major advantage in the use of GnRH agonist is the complete elimination of the preovulatory LH surge; in addition to preventing cycle cancellations due to premature ovulation, the use of GnRH agonist has permitted to dramatically reduce endocrine monitoring and its related costs. Nevertheless, clomiphene citrate action is dependent upon pituitary sensitivity to endogenous GnRH, thus rendering thus drug ineffective during GnRH agonist administration.

GnRH agonist regimens

The administration of GnRH agonist initially stimulates endogenous gonadotropin secretion; however, pituitary desensitization and profound suppression of LH (and to a lesser extent, of FSH) serum levels eventually ensues[2,3]. The goal of GnRH agonist in COS is to prevent the spontaneous preovulatory LH surge triggered by mounting levels of estrogens stimulated by exogenous gonadotropins. Given the early stimulatory action of GnRH agonist, these compounds must be started several days before ovarian follicle maturation is achieved.

Numerous variations in GnRH agonist regimens, route of administration, and dosages have been proposed in recent years. Administration regimens can be summarized as follows[4]:

a. Long regimens. The GnRH agonist is started in the mid-luteal phase of the cycle preceding ovulation induction (or earlier) and continued until ovulation is triggered with hCG. Once ovarian suppression is confirmed by low estradiol (E_2) levels exogenous gonadotropins are started; at this time endogenous gonadotropins are suppressed and follicle stimulation depends almost entirely on exogenous gonadotropins.

b. Short (or flare-up) regimens. The GnRH agonist is started in the early follicular phase of the COS cycle concomitantly with exogenous gonadotropins and continued until hCG administration. The rationale of this regimen is that the "flare" effect of the GnRH agonist on FSH secretion would synergize with exogenous gonadotropin stimulation and thus facilitate COS, thereby reducing exogenous gonadotropin dose requirements. Nevertheless, it was shown that the degree of folliculogenesis achieved with the short regimen is lower than with the long regimen in spite of higher follicular phase FSH levels[5]. This effect may be due to the increased intrafollicular androgen levels encountered in short regimens[6] that may cause follicle atresia and thus reduce oocyte yield[7].

c. Ultrashort regimen. Also in this type of regimen the GnRH agonist is begun in the early follicular phase of the COS cycle but it is discontinued after only three days[8]. This treatment modality counts on prolonged pituitary desensitization beyond the short period of GnRH agonist administration.

d. Preparatory regimen. The GnRH agonist is started in the mid-luteal phase of the cycle preceding COS (like in the long regimen) but it is discontinued when exogenous gonadotropins are begun[9]. Also in this case, it is postulated that partial pituitary desensitization can be maintained for several days following GnRH agonist discontinuation. Nevertheless, such a long lasting effect of only a few days of GnRH agonist administration was never proven neither for the ultrashort nor for the preparatory regimen and thus doubts persist regarding the full clinical efficacy of these approaches.

Over the last decade the long GnRH agonist regimen has prevailed over different administration schedules and is now adopted in over 90% of COS cycles for AR worldwide. The reason of this success are manifold[4]:

a. Convenience in patients scheduling: treatment can be started at any time after pituitary desensitization is achieved regardless of spontaneous menstrual cyclicity of patients.

b. Standardization of baseline patient conditions. As pituitary-ovarian quiescence is achieved in most patients by the time COS is started, more homogeneous baseline conditions and a more consistent response to treatment can be envisioned in these patients.

c. Improved folliculogenesis. The majority of comparison studies found a significantly greater number of preovulatory follicles and an improved oocyte yield in the long over the short regimen. As follicular phase FSH levels are more elevated in the short regimen[6] other endocrine mechanisms appear to prevent the purported synergism between GnRH agonist stimulated pituitary FSH secretion and exogenous gonadotropin administration. One possible explanation of this apparent discrepancy is that, as GnRH agonist in the flare-up mode stimulate both pituitary gonadotropins, LH will excessively stimulate theca cell androgen production that in turn may cause follicle atresia. In support of this hypothesis we found that follicular fluid testosterone levels are significantly higher in patients treated with the short GnRH agonist regimen than in those treated without GnRH agonist or, even more significantly, with a long GnRH agonist regimen[6].

GnRH antagonists

Although GnRH agonist and GnRH antagonist development started concurrently in the mid 1970s, synthesis of these compounds progressed at different speed. Because of the relative simplicity of polypeptide chain modifications required for GnRH agonist these compounds were developed and became clinically available in a relatively short timespan. The GnRH agonist Buserelin was registered in Europe in the late 1970s; conversely, Cetrorelix will be the first GnRH antagonist on the market and this will occur in 1999, i.e. more than twenty years following Buserelin registration.

GnRH antagonist are characterized by a more complex structure and more extensive modifications of the native GnRH aminoacid sequence, particularly in the early 3 aminoacid portion responsible for pituitary receptor binding and activation. GnRH antagonist administration causes an immediate block of gonadotropins secretion; thus LH and FSH levels immediately decline after GnRH antagonist without the flare-up effect typical of GnRH agonist. GnRH antagonist are also more effective than GnRH agonist in suppressing FSH secretion when administered at high dosages.

The capacity of GnRH antagonist of immediately suppressing pituitary gonadotropin secretion was successfully exploited for devising alternative COS regimens. GnRH antagonist are usually administered after several days of gonadotropin administration and are highly effective to prevent the spontaneous preovulatory LH surge or block it if already initiated[10,11]. Two types of GnRH antagonist regimens have been tested so far. The more commonly used low dose regimen consists of starting GnRH antagonist (e.g. Cetrorelix 0.25 mg daily) after about six days of gonadotropin stimulation and continuing it until the time of hCG administration. Alternatively, a high single dose of GnRH antagonist (e.g. Cetrorelix 3.0 mg) can be administered towards the end of gonadotropin COS (around day 9) and repeated after two days, if needed.

Both these regimens appear to be effective for COS in AR programs and are expected to be implemented clinically on a wide scale once GnRH antagonist are registered. Whether or not GnRH antagonist will totally replace GnRH agonist in AR program is still the subject of debate; potential limits of GnRH antagonist administered with the regimens previously outlined include:

- reduced practicality of patient scheduling;
- possible reductions of folliculogenesis and oocyte yield;
- excessive suppression of endogenous gonadotropins.

Additional studies will be needed to further assess efficacy of GnRH antagonist in COS and the possibility of administering them in different regimens.

Exogenous gonadotropins

The preparations and regimens of exogenous gonadotropins available for ovulation induction have also extensively changed in the last two decades. Three major changes have occurred in this pharmaceutical field:

1. Development of urinary gonadotropin preparations (menotropins) with progressive reduction in the content of LH. While the original menotropins (Pergonal, Humegon) contained the same LH and FSH unit amounts (75 IU each per ampoule), later preparations were progressively depleted of LH (25-35 IU per ampoule); the introduction of purified FSH (pFSH, <1.0 IU LH per ampoule) and of highly purified FSH (HP FSH, <0.1 IU LH per ampoule) virtually eliminated LH activity from these menotropins preparations.

2. Reduction of proteinaceous material contamination from menotropin preparations. The original menotropin preparations contained large amounts of pharmacological inactive contaminants that were linked with rare allergic-type reactions[12]. The newer HP menotropin preparations are virtually devoid of these contaminants and thus associated with an allergenic profile comparable to synthetically produced gonadotropins.

3. Synthesis of gonadotropins with recombinant DNA techniques. These synthetic procedures have allowed the development and production of pure gonadotropin preparations (both LH and FSH) totally devoid of nonspecific activities. While recombinant human FSH (r-hFSH) is currently commercially

available and widely used, r-hLH has not been registered yet. Potential applications of r-hLH include replacement of hCG as ovulation triggering agent and supplementation of r-hFSH ovulation induction in hypogonadotropic conditions.

Pathophysiologic correlates of clinical efficacy

Ovulation induction for AR has achieved high levels of efficacy regardless of the specific COS regimen chosen. Nevertheless, several physiologic and pathophysiologic features of the reproductive system have important therapeutic implications and are valuable to optimize and enhance efficacy and ovulation induction safety.

The trend in the combined use of gonadotropin preparations progressively devoid of LH activity and of GnRH analogs that suppress endogenous gonadotropin secretion has resulted in an overall hypo-LH follicular phase milieu. This development is at least in part related to the perception that LH is a "bad" gonadotropin for follicular and oocyte maturation. While extensive evidence exists regarding a detrimental role on reproductive function of tonically elevated LH secretion particularly in polycystic ovary syndrome (PCOS) patients[13], there are no indications that this may apply to LH-containing menotropins.

The administration of moderate hMG dosages (150 IU LH and 150 IU FSH) to both normal and PCOS women caused mild and mostly nonsignificant short time serum LH elevations; by 24h LH levels returned to baseline values[14]. Longer-term hMG administration in PCOS actually results in a progressive decline of peripheral LH levels; this effect is likely due to the negative feed back effect on the pituitary of the rising levels of FSH-stimulated E_2 and inhibin. A corollary of these findings is that virtually no difference between hMG and FSH-only menotropins could be detected in any of the studies in which these preparations were compared for PCOS ovulation induction[15-18].

Conversely, there is evidence that moderate LH activity in gonadotropin preparation may be advantageous for ovulation induction. LH is indispensable to stimulate theca cell androgens that are subsequently transformed into estrogens in granulosa cells. Thus, low or insufficient LH stimulation may result in reduced estrogen production. Estrogens in turn exert positive effects on the oocyte cytoplasm[19,20] and oolemma[20,21], and on embryo maturation[22]. Reduced follicular fluid E_2 levels are associated with a poor outcome of in-vitro fertilization[23].

When treating patients with hypogonadotropic hypogonadism LH activity is needed to optimize the outcome of ovulation induction. When compared to the use of pFSH or r-hFSH alone, hMG administration[24] or supplementation with r-hLH[25] permits to reduce exogenous FSH dose and the duration of stimulation, to increase preovulatory E_2 levels and the ovulation rate, and to improve oocyte fertilization and pregnancy rates.

As it is likely that relatively low serum LH concentration (1-2 IU/L) are sufficient to provide adequate ovarian support, several approaches may be appropriate to produce sufficient LH input:

1. The most obvious approach to provide an LH stimulus is to use hMG regardless of the stimulation regimen employed. Unfortunately in many countries hMG is no longer available or difficult to obtain.

2. Once it becomes clinically available the use of r-hLH could be advocated in combination with FSH-only menotropins or r-hFSH. Although the proper r-hLH dose for COS has not been determined yet, optimal results in HH ovulation induction are obtained with 75 IU of r-hLH per day.

3. Along the same line, LH activity in ovulation induction may be supplemented with the administration of low-dose hCG.

4. Finally, the use of low-dose GnRH agonist or GnRH antagonist regimens provides less profound endogenous LH suppression and is associated with a better overall outcome of ovulation induction. Evidence of better outcome of lower dose GnRH analog regimens is most convincing in the case of GnRH-ant. A recently completed dose finding study of the GnRH antagonist Ganirelix clearly indicated that combining r-hFSH stimulation with the higher Ganirelix dosages (i.e. a condition likely to virtually eliminate ovarian LH input) was associated with significantly reduced preovulatory E_2 levels and pregnancy rates as well as high miscarriage rates[26].

Conclusions

Ovulation induction regimens for AR techniques have dramatically evolved in the last two decades. New, more refined gonadotropin preparations have become available over this period and new developments in this pharmaceutical field are likely in the near future. GnRH agonist have become an integral and unreplaceable part of these regimens and their use has brought about marked improvement in the outcome of COS. The near availability of GnRH antagonist will permit to further improve choice and flexibility of ovulation induction regimens. Finally, special attention will have to be devoted to the beneficial role that exogenous and/or endogenous LH activity may play in ovulation induction regimens and to the possible strategies needed to therapeutically optimize the role of this often overlooked gonadotropin.

References

1. Dodson W.C., Hughes C.L., Whitesides D.B., Haney A.F.: The effect of leuprolide acetate on ovulation induction with human menopausal gonadotropins in polycystic ovary syndrome. *J. Clin. Endocrinol. Metab.*, 65:95-100,1987.
2. Filicori M., Flamigni C.: GnRH agonists and antagonists. Current clinical status. *Drugs*, 35:63-82,1988.
3. Filicori M.: Gonadotrophin-releasing hormone agonists. A guide to use and selection. *Drugs*, 48:41-58,1994.
4. Filicori M.: Clinical review 81: Gonadotropin-releasing hormone analogs in ovulation induction: current status and perspectives. *J. Clin. Endocrinol. Metab.*, 81:2413-6,1996.
5. Tan S.L., Kingsland C., Campbell S., Mills C., Bradfield J., Alexander N., et al.: The long protocol of administration of gonadotropin-releasing hormone agonist is superior to the short protocol for ovarian stimulation for in vitro fertilization. *Fertil. Steril.*, 57:810-814,1992.
6. Filicori M., Flamigni C., Cognigni G.E., Falbo A., Arnone R., Capelli M., et al.: Different gonadotropin and leuprorelin ovulation induction regimens markedly affect follicular fluid hormone levels and folliculogenesis. *Fertil. Steril.*, 65:387-393,1996.
7. Louvet J.P., Harman S.M., Schrieber J.R., Ross G.T.: Evidence of a role of adrogens in follicular maturation. *Endocrinology*, 97:366-372,1975.
8. Ron El R., Herman A., Golan A., Soffer Y., Nachum H., Caspi E.: Ultrashort gonadotropin-releasing hormone agonist (GnRH-a) protocol in comparison with the long-acting GnRH-a protocol and menotropin alone. *Fertil. Steril.*, 58:1164-1168,1992.
9. Pantos K., Meimeth Damianaki T., Vaxevanoglou T., Kapetanakis E.: Prospective study of a modified gonadotropin-releasing hormone agonist long protocol in an in vitro fertilization program. *Fertil. Steril.*, 61:709-713,1994.
10. Dubourdieu S., Charbonnel B., D'Acremont M.F., Carreau S., Spitz I.M., Bouchard P.: Effect of administration of a gonadotropin-releasing hormone (GnRH) antagonist (Nal-Glu) during the periovulatory period: the luteinizing hormone surge requires secretion of GnRH. *J. Clin. Endocrinol. Metab.*, 78:343-747,1994.
11. Olivennes F., Fanchin R., Bouchard P., de Ziegler D., Taieb J., Selva J., et al.: The single or dual administration of the gonadotropin-releasing hormone antagonist Cetrorelix in an in vitro fertilization-embryo transfer program. *Fertil. Steril.*, 62:468-476,1994.
12. Biffoni M., Marcucci I., Ythier A., Eshkol A.: Effects of urinary gonadotro-

pin preparations on human in-vitro immune function. *Hum. Reprod.*, 13:2430-2434,1998.

13. Shoham Z., Jacobs H.S., Insler V.: Luteinizing hormone: its role, mechanism of action, and detrimental effects when hypersecreted during the follicular phase. *Fertil. Steril.*, 59:1153-1161,1993.
14. Anderson R.E., Cragun J.M., Chang R.J., Stanczyk F.Z., Lobo R.A.: A pharmacodynamic comparison of human urinary follicle-stimulating hormone and human menopausal gonadotropin in normal women and polycystic ovary syndrome. *Fertil. Steril.*, 52:216-220,1989.
15. Tanbo T., Dale P.O., Kjekshus E., Haug E., Abyholm T.: Stimulation with human menopausal gonadotropin versus follicle-stimulating hormone after pituitary suppression in polycystic ovarian syndrome. *Fertil. Steril.*, 53:798-803,1990.
16. Larsen T., Larsen J.F., Schioler V., Bostofte E., Felding C.: Comparison of urinary human follicle-stimulating hormone and human menopausal gonadotropin for ovarian stimulation in polycystic ovarian syndrome. *Fertil. Steril.*, 53:426-431,1990.
17. Sagle M.A., Hamilton F.D., Kiddy D.S., Franks S.: A comparative, randomized study of low-dose human menopausal gonadotropin and follicle-stimulating hormone in women with polycystic ovarian syndrome. *Fertil. Steril.*, 55:56-60,1991.
18. Venturoli S., Paradisi R., Fabbri R., Magrini O., Porcu E., Flamigni C.: Comparison between human urinary follicle-stimulating hormone and human menopausal gonadotropin treatment in polycystic ovary. *Obstet. Gynecol.*, 63:6-11,1984.
19. Yoshimura Y., Wallach E.E.: Studies of the mechanism(s) of mammalian ovulation. *Fertil. Steril.*, 47:22-34,1987.
20. Tesarik J., Mendoza C.: Nongenomic effects of 17 beta-estradiol on maturing human oocytes: relationship to oocyte developmental potential. *J. Clin. Endocrinol. Metab.*, 80:1438-1443,1995.
21. Palermo G.D., Alikani M., Bertoli M., Colombero L.T., Moy F., Cohen J., et al.: Oolemma characteristics in relation to survival and fertilization patterns of oocytes treated by intracytoplasmic sperm injection. *Hum. Reprod.*, 11:172-176,1996.
22. Weston A.M., Zelinski-Wooten M.B., Hutchison J.S., Stouffer R.L., Wolf D.P.: Developmental potential of embryos produced by in-vitro fertilization from gonadotrophin-releasing hormone antagonist-treated macaques stimulated with recombinant human follicle stimulating hormone alone or in combination with luteinizing hormone. *Hum. Reprod.*, 11:608-613,1996.
23. Loumaye E., Engrand P., Howles C.M., O'Dea L.: Assessment of the role

of serum luteinizing hormone and estradiol response to follicle-stimulating hormone on in vitro fertilization treatment outcome. *Fertil. Steril.*, 67:889-899,1997.
24. Couzinet B., Lestrat N., Brailly S., Forest M., Schaison G.: Stimulation of ovarian follicular maturation with pure follicle-stimulating hormone in women with gonadotropin deficiency. *J. Clin. Endocrinol. Metab.*, 66:552-556,1988.
25. The European recombinant human LH study group: Recombinant human luteinizing hormone (LH) to support recombinant human follicle-stimulating hormone (FSH)-induced follicular development in LH- and FSH-deficient anovulatory women: a dose-finding study. *J. Clin. Endocrinol. Metab.*, 83:1507-1514,1998.
26. The ganirelix dose-finding study group. A double-blind, randomised, dose-finding study to assess the efficacy of the GnRH antagonist Ganirelix (Org 37462) to prevent premature LH surges in women undergoing controlled ovarian hyperstimulation with recombinant FSH (Puregon). *Hum. Reprod.*, 13:3023-3031, 1998.

The Role of Luteinizing Hormone
in Folliculogenesis
and Ovulation Induction, pp. 155-172
Editor M. Filicori

Use of Recombinant FSH in Assisted Reproduction

K. Diedrich and R. Felberbaum

Department of Obstetrics and Gynecology, Medical University of Lübeck (Germany)

Abstract. *While in the early times of IVF only the natural cycle was regarded as being able to allow the aspiration of a mature metaphase II - oocyte to be fertilized* in vitro, *in the meantime controlled ovarian hyperstimulation (COH) using human menopausal gonadotrophins (HMG) became a well established therapeutic attitude. In combination with GnRH-agonists used for prevention of premature luteinization COH with HMG granted an acceptable therapeutic outcome and favourable pregnancy rates. Preparations of HMG normally contain equivalent FSH- and LH-activity, which in some indications like PCOD may be not intended. Other disadvantages of HMG may be the necessity of intramuscular injection, the dependency on urine donors and the high quantity of congener urinary proteins which may be responsable for adverse events after administration. Nowadays highly purified urinary FSH preparations as well as preparations of recombinant FSH are available, the latter one being totally free of any LH-activity. After having fully isolated the α- and β- gene for FSH and introduction of these genes into a mammalian cell line (Chinese Hamster Ovary cell line [CHO]) it was possible to produce genetically engineered, biologically active FSH. Rec. FSH can be produced in huge amounts independent of any donors, its preparations are absolutely pure and of consistent quality and can be administered subcutaneously. Rec. FSH has been proven to be highly efficient as well in COH for ART as for monofollicular development and ovulation induction for conception* in vivo. *Only in WHO-I patients the absence of any LH-activity may lead to follicular growth, but to insufficient estradiol secretion due to the lack of androgen precursors. In the combination with GnRH-agonists or -antagonists there is sufficient LH present to provide a satisfactory estradiol production. Patients compliance and comfort in administration are excellent. However, the discussion about differences in the therapeutic outcome comparing urinary and recombinant compounds is still going on. Huge metaanalysis presented to document a benefit in favour of rec. FSH showed an important bias. Even in an indication like PCOD with its elevated LH levels advantages of rec. FSH could not be proven in the sense of evidence based medicine until now. Rec. LH, recently developed seems to be a* *compound in search for its clinical indication. On the other hand rec. FSH has increased the costs for COH in ART tremendously. This means a very important burden for national health services as well as for patients in countries where ART is not covered by the health authorities. Arguments in favour of a higher safety standard seems to be fairly weak, as urinary compounds had been presented for more than 15 years as safe products. Probably softer stimulation protocols like Clomiphene Citrate in combination with rec. FSH and GnRH-antagonists or very low stimulation for ART in the natural cycle, using also GnRH-antagonists for prevention of spontanous ovulation may help to find the right place for rec. FSH within ART.*

Key words. FSH, recombinant FSH, controlled ovarian hyperstimulation.

Introduction

While in the early years of IVF, when Louise Brown was born in 1978 only the natural cycle was believed to allow the retrieval of an mature metaphase II oocyte for fertilization *in vitro*, it could be shown quite early that superovulation, as having been described in the animal, was also possible in the human[1-4]. The principle of controlled ovarian hyperstimulation (COH), using antiestrogens like Clomiphen Citrate, or mainly human gonadotrophins had an overwhelming impact on assisted reproduction worldwide. The possibility to rescue several oocytes from their destination to atresia, to be able to aspirate them and by that to increase as well the fertilization rates in vitro as the number of embryos to be replaced in utero was one of the most important developments of the last 20 years, leading to acceptable pregnancy rates. By introducing GnRH agonists into controlled ovarian hyperstimulation (COH), the premature luteinization as major drawback of a stimulation with hMG only could be avoided almost completely. Especially the "long protocol", aiming at complete desensitization of the pituitary gland before starting the stimulatory therapy has become a widely accepted treatment of first choice[5]. More oocytes to be rescued meant more oocytes to be fertilized *in vitro* and more embryos to be transferred in each attempt at treatment. This greatly raised the success rate in terms of pregnancies achieved.

Recombinant gonadotropins

Recent advances in bioengineering made it possible to produce a recombinant preparation of human FSH *in vitro*. As FSH needs to be glycosylated for its biological activity, recombinant FSH is produced by genetically engineered Chinese hamster ovary [CHO] cells, in which the genes coding for the α- and ß subunits are inserted[6]. Pharmaceutical peparations of urinary human gonadotrophins (HMG) contain a mixture of FSH and LH and are of low specific activity (about 100 - 150 IU FSH/mg protein). More than 95% of protein content consists of non-specific co-purified urinay proteins. Rec. FSH instead is totally free of any LH activity and of extremely high purity (mean specific activity 10.000 IU/mg of protein). It is at least debatable whether this high purity may have clinical advantages concerning the discussed improved batch-to-batch consistency due to permanent control of the FSH isoform profile, contrasting with current HMG and urinary hFSH preparations[7,8]. Recent case reports suggesting that copurified urinary proteins could lead to adverse immune reaction are a little bit puzzling, as for more than fifteen years urinary preparations have been thought to be absolutely safe. Due to its high purity rec. FSH shows a bioavailability of 75% both after subcutan administration and after intramuscular injection. This decreases patients burden to some extent[9].

Recombinant FSH in COH for IVF-ET

It could be demonstrated that – with the exception of WHO I patients – in spite of downregulation of the pituitary gland by a GnRH agonist endogenous LH secretion is sufficient to allow satisfactory ovarian stimulation by pure rec. FSH. In gonadotropin-deficient WHO I patients the daily administration of pure FSH may lead to multiple follicular growth up to the preovulatory stage, but serum and follicular fluid steroid concentrations will remain very low[10]. In a metaanalysis of 8 studies comprising 592 patients controlled ovarian hyperstimulation with FSH revealed significant higher pregnancy rates in comparison to the use of hMG[11-12]. In another metaanalysis performed by Out et al. three prospective, multicenter randomized comparative trials were combined. 697 infertile women receiving recombinant FSH were compared to 463 women receiving hMG or urinary FSH, all of them undergoing one cycle of controlled ovarian hyperstimulation for IVF-ET. In the presented analysis the ongoing pregnancy rate was 22.9% for recombinant FSH and 17.9% for urinary gonadotropins. This 5% treatment difference was statistically significant[13]. However, only in two of these three studies a GnRH-agonist was used in a long protocol setting, both comparing recombinant and urinary FSH. In the third study rec. FSH was compared with hMG without the use of any GnRH-analogue in both groups. These differences in study design may indicate an important problem within metaanalyses as different studies with different design and not at all comparable results are mixed together. Nevertheless metaanalyses are used increasingly in reproductive medicine to synthesize research[14]. Another major obstacle in assessing the value of metaanalysis is the socalled publication bias. True differences may be overestimated because negative results are likely not to have been published as admitted by the authors themselves[13]. Other studies have not demonstrated as clear differences in outcome between the two gonadotropins. Compared to urinary highly purified FSH, rec.FSH showed no differences regarding follicular maturation in the long agonistic protocol[15].

The fact that two recombinant FSH preparations have been commercialized (follitropin α - Gonal F, Ares Serono, Geneva, Switzerland and follitropin ß - Puregon, NV Organon, Oss, The Netherlands) may indicate that these two compounds may be different due to slightly different purification procedures. However, it is still unproven that these differences may lead to different pharmacological effects. There has been no comparative study using both recombinant FSH preparations so far. It is at least remarkable that in another prospective randomised study, comparing follitropin ß with urinary FSH significantly more cumulus-oocyte complexes and mature oocytes were retrieved from those patients who received rec.FSH[16].

Recombinant FSH in combination with GnRH-antagonists

The fourth generation GnRH-antagonists Cetrorelix and Ganirelix are tested at present time within the frame of clinical phase-II and phase III - studies in combination with recombinant FSH. The effectiveness of rec. FSH within

TABLE 1 - *Follicular development, results of Ovum pick up (OPU) and IVF-results after controlled ovarian hyperstimulation (COH) with rec. FSH (Gonal-F/follitropin alpha) or urinary FSH in combination with buserelin acetate (200 µg/d s.s.) according to the "long" protocol[15].*

	rec.FSH	*uFSH*	*Significance*
Patients (n)	60	63	
Estradiol concentration on day of HCG (pg/ml)	1575	2192	0,0007
Oocytes retrieved	9,3	10,7	NS
Fertilized oocytes	5,6	6,5	NS
Cleaved embryos	5	6,1	NS
clin. pregnancies/cycle (%)	20	16	NS

controlled ovarian hyperstimulation according to the long protocol has been proven. Even after down regulation of the pituitary gland endogenous LH-secretion seems to be sufficient for normal ovarian sexual steroids biosynthesis. However extreme suppression of LH-secretion by high doses of GnRH-antagonists could cause problems according to the two-cells/two gonadotrophin hypothesis of follicular estrogen production[17]. Causing a situation very similar to WHO-I infertile patients ovarian stimulation with pure FSH, depleted of any LH-activity could induce follicular growth in the absence of any estrogen secretion, as having been described for these patients[10]. It is the merit of the prospective, multicentric double blinded dose finding phase II – study with Ganirelix to have elucidated this question and having demonstrated the correctness of the two cell – two gonadotrophin theory. In this study Ganirelix was administered according to the multiple dose "Lübeck protocol" in six different dosages (0.0625 mg/day, 0.125 mg/day, 0.25 mg/day, 0,5 mg/day, 1 mg/day and 2 mg/day). While in the lower dosages estradiol secretion was normal and sufficient, injecting 2 mg Ganirelix s.c. per day almost no increase of the estradiol secretion could be seen. In some cases even the follicles did not grow, an observation that still awaits its scientific explanation. The treatment outcome in the 0.25 mg - group was an overwhelming success

TABLE 2 - *Follicular development, results of Ovum pick up (OPU) and IVF-results after controlled ovarian hyperstimulation (COH) with rec.FSH (Puregon/follitropin beta) or urinary FSH in combination with buserelin acetate (intranasal application) according to the "long" protocol*[16].

	rec.FSH	*uFSH*	*Significance*
Patients (n)	585	396	
Total FSH dose (IU)	2138	2385	< 0,0001
Duration of FSH (days)	10,7	11,3	< 0,0001
Estradiol concentration on day of HCG (pg/ml)	6084	5179	< 0,0001
Oocytes retrieved (n)	10,8	9	< 0,0001
High quality embryos	3,11	2,61	0,003
Ongoing pregnancies/cycle (%)			
Fresh	22,2	18,2	NS
Fresh + cryo	25,6	20,4	0,05

showing a clinical pregnancy rate of 40.3% per transfer. Increasing the dosage of Ganirelix let the pregnancy rates drop and the abortion rates rise. Thus 0.25 mg was defined as the minimal effective dose to be administered according to the multiple dose protocol. However, we have to wait, if this obvious great success can be repeated in the ongoing phase III - study, using 0.25 mg Ganirelix per day[18].

Recombinant FSH and costs – a matter of debate

The development of recombinant gonadotropins and their introduction onto the market entailed an important scientific advance, while treatment costs were increased tremendously. Although that lowering the price for these compounds would be expected to replace the urinary ones almost totally, recombinant gonadotropins remain extremely expensive. Overall, the most promising aspect of introducing GnRH antagonists into COH may be the possibility of making this treatment less aggressive and much softer than an agonistic long protocol, using old-fashioned schemes of stimulation such as clomiphene citrate or CC in combination with hMG and/or rec FSH[19]. Probably softer stimulation protocols like Clomiphene Citrate in combination with rec. FSH and GnRH-antagonists or very low stimulation for ART in the natural cycle, using also GnRH-antagonists for prevention of spontanous ovulation may help to find the right place for rec. FSH within ART[20].

References

1. Steptoe P.C., Edwards R.G.: Birth after reimplantation of a human embryo. *Lancet*, II:366, 1978.
2. Edwards R.G.: Test tube babies. *Nature*, 293:253-256.
3. Trounson A.O., Leeton J.F., Wood C., Webb J., Wood J.: Pregnancies in humans by fertilization in vitro and embryo transfer in the controlled ovulatory cycle. *Science*, 212:681-682, 1981.
4. Trounson A.O.: In vitro fertilization at Monash University, Melbourne, Australia. In: Crosignani P.G., Rubin B.L. (eds), *In vitro fertilization and embryo transfer*. Academic Press, New York, pp. 315-322.
5. Wildt L., Diedrich K., van der ven H., Al-Hasani S., Hubner H., Klasen R.: Ovarian hyperstimulation for in vitro fertilization controlled by GnRH agnist administered in combination with hMG. *Hum. Reprod.*, 1:15-19, 1986.
6. Chappel S., Kelton C., Nugent N.: Expression of human gonadotropins by recombinant DNA methods. In: Genazzi A.R., Petraglia F. (eds), *Proceedings of the 3rd World Congress on Gynaecological Endocrinology*. Carnforth, The

Partenon Publishing Group, pp. 179-184, 1992.

7. Out. H.J., Mannaerts B., Driessen A., et al.: Recombinant follicle stimulating hormone (rFSH); Puregon) in assisted reproduction: More oocytes, more pregnancies, Results from five comparative studies. *Hum. Reprod. Update*, 2:162-171, 1996.
8. Rector N.A., Markusen T.E., Stone B.A., Marrs R.P.: Number and quality of oocytes with induction of multiple follliculogenesis in women and in mice with different lots of human menopausal gonadotropins. *Fertil. Steril.*, 60:1082-1087, 1993.
9. Loumaye E., Campbell R., Salat-Baroux J.: Human follicle stimulating hormone produced by recombinant DNA technology: a review for clinicians. *Hum. Reprod. Update*, 1:188-199, 1995.
10. Schoot D.C., Coelingh-Bennink H.J.T., Mannaerts B., et al.: Human recombinant follicle-stimulating hormone induces growth of preovulatory follicles without concomitant increase in androgen and estrogen biosynthesis in a women with isolated gonadotropin deficiency. *J. Clin. Endocrinol. Metab.*, 74:1471-1473, 1992.
11. Daya S., Gunby J., Hughes E.G. et al.: Follicle stimulating hormone versus human menopausal gonadotropin for in vitro fertilization cycles: a meta analysis. *Fertil. Steril.*, 64:347-354, 1995.
12. Daya S., Gunby J., Hughes E.G. et al.: Randomized controlled trial of follicle stimulating hormone versus human menopausal gonadotropin in in vitro fertilization. *Hum. Reprod.*, 10:1392-1396, 1995.
13. Out H.J., Driessen S., Mannaerts B., Coelingh-Bennink H.J.T.: Recombinant follicle-stimulating hormone (follitropin beta, Puregon) yields higher pregnancy rates in in vitro fertilization than urinary gonadotrophins. *Fertil. Steril.*, 68:138-142, 1997.
14. Hughes E.G., Sagle M.A., Fedorkow D.M., Koppel P. van de, Daya S., Collins J.A.: The routine use of gonadotropin-releasing hormone agonists prior to in vitro fertilization and gamete intrafallopian transfer: a meta-analysis of randomised controlled trials. *Fertil. Steril.*, 58:888-896, 1992.
15. Recombinant human FSH study group: Clinical assessment of recombinant human follicle-stimulating hormone in stimulating ovarian follicular development before in vitro fertilization. *Fertil. Steril.*, 63:77-86, 1995.
16. Out H.J., Mannaerts B., Driessen S., et al.: A prospective, randomized, assessorblind, multicentre study comparing recombinant and urinary follicle stimulating hormone (Puregon versus Metrodin) in in vitro fertilization. *Hum. Reprod.*, 10:2534-2540, 1995.
17. Hillier S.G., Whitelaw P.F., Smyth C.D.: Follicular estrogen synthesis: the "two cell, two gonadotropin" model revisited. *Mol. Cell. Endocrinol.*, 100:51-

54, 1994.

18. The Ganirelix dose-finding study group: A double-blind, randomized, dose finding study to assess the efficacy of the gonadotrophin-releasing hormone antagonist Ganirelix (Org 37462) to prevent premature luteinizing hormone surges in women undergoing ovarian stimulation with recombinant follicle stimulating hormone (Puregon). *Hum. Reprod.*, 13:3023-3031, 1998.
19. Felberbaum R.E., Ludwig M., Diedrich K.: Are we on the verge of a new era in ART? *Hum. Reprod.*, 13:1778-1780, 1998.
20. Olivennes F., Rongières-Bertrand C., Righini C., Fanchin R., Taieb J., Bouchard P., Frydman R.: The use in IVF-embryo transfer of a new GnRH antagonist (Cetrorelix) in natural cycles associated with minimal stimulation. *Hum. Reprod.*, 13(Abstract book 1):195, 1998.

The Role of Luteinizing Hormone
in Folliculogenesis
and Ovulation Induction, pp. 173-188
Editor M. Filicori

Clinical Outcome of *In-vitro* Fertilization: hMG vs. Purified FSH

L. Westergaard

Fertility Clinic, Odense University Hospital, Odense C (Denmark)

Abstract. *Both LH and FSH are required for normal follicular development and oestrogen production in women. Although use of recombinant human FSH – devoid of LH activity – for ovarian stimulation of women with hypogonadotrophic hypogonadism allows for preovulatory follicular development with very low oestradiol production, the reproductive outcome will be compromised. Conversely, increased levels of LH in the circulation also seem to compromise the reproductive outcome in women with normal menstrual cycle as well as women treated with exogenous gonadotropins. Suppressing pituitary gonadotropin secretion with GnRH analogues during stimulation with exogenous gonadotrophins has improved the success rates of IVF significantly. In normogonadotropic women low levels of resting LH seem sufficient to support follicular and oocyte development and oestradiol production, as evidenced by the good results of IVF treatment when using "pure" FSH (urine-derived or human recombinant) in combination with GnRH-a down-regulation. Indeed, it has been proposed, that the LH contained in the classical hMG preparations may be detrimental to the outcome of IVF, and that "pure" FSH preparations should replace hMG for ovarian stimulation in normogonadotropic women. Evidence based on controlled clinical trials comparing the effects of FSH and hMG in GnRH-a down-regulated women do not support this notion. Although most clinical trials find equivalency between FSH and hMG, some recent data indicate that there may be a substantial subgroup of normogonadotropic women, whose endogenous LH secretion is so profoundly suppressed by a standard GnRH-a treatment, that the outcome of IVF is compromised, when treated with "pure" FSH. Whether these women would benefit from treatment with hMG or rec. FSH combined with rec. LH remains to be proven in future prospective, randomized trials.*

Key words. Purified FSH, LH, HMG, GnRH agonist down-regulation, IVF outcome.

Introduction

During the natural menstrual cycle a finely tuned and ever changing balance between follicle stimulating hormone (FSH) and luteinizing hormone (LH) secures the proper growth, maturation and ovulation of only one follicle and its oocyte.

According to the now proven two-cell two-gonadotrophin concept of ovarian oestradiol synthesis circulating LH stimulates androgen production of the theca interna cells, which upon transfer to the avascular granulosa cell layer is aromatized into oestradiol under the influence of FSH[1]. In preovulatory follicles LH is also capable of inducing oestradiol synthesis[2]. In addition, FSH and LH may also – via locally produced mediators – influence other aspects of follicular development, e.g. oocyte nuclear and cytoplasmic maturation and subsequent embryo quality[3-5].

Disturbance of the normal balance between FSH and LH may result in infertility due to anovulation with amenorrhoea, affect fertilization of the ovulated oocyte negatively or cause poor development of the implanted embryo with increased risk of early pregnancy loss.

Exogenous gonadotropins have for the last 35 years been used successfully in the treatment of anovulatory infertility due to gonadotropin imbalances. The introduction of IVF treatment boosted the use of exogenous gonadotrophins for controlled ovarian hyperstimulation, also in normogonadotropic women. Despite the widespread use of gonadotropins, however, the precise gonadotropin requirements of the developing ovarian follicle have not yet been established and especially the role of LH in this process has been controversial[6].

Ovarian Stimulation with Gonadotropins in IVF Treatment

Although the first human baby born after conception in vitro resulted from oocyte aspiration in a natural, unstimulated cycle[7], it soon became clear that increasing the number of mature oocytes by controlled ovarian hyperstimulation and ovulation induction improved the success rates of IVF significantly[8]. Therefore, since the earliest days of IVF human menopausal gonadotrophin (hMG) has been administered to normogonadotropic women to induce multiple follicular growth in order to maximize the yield of oocytes for fertilization *in vitro*. However, these stimulation methods possessed two major drawbacks, which have been ascribed to effects of LH: 1) due to frequent occurrence of an untimely, spontaneous LH surge the outcome was often jeopardized; 2) there is evidence to assume, that increased tonic levels of LH in the circulation during the follicular phase of the cycle are associated with reduced rates of fertilization and implantation and increased miscarriage rates. This association seems to be valid for patients with polycystic ovarian syndrome (PCOS) as well as for women with normal ovaries and cycles, and was found not only in women undergoing treatment with ovarian stimulation, but also in women achieving spontaneous pregnancy[9-12]. Although the exact mechanism by which increased levels of LH in the follicular phase of the cycle reduce fertility still remain unclear, it is generally believed that LH induces a premature resumption of meiosis, leading to ovulation/retrieval of postmature or "aged" oocytes with a reduced capacity to fertilize and to undergo normal embryonal development[13]. In addition, it has been proposed that increased LH levels by induction of an abnormally high androgen production by the theca cells may lead to a reduced implantation potential of the possible embryos[14].

During the 1980's two measures were introduced in order to deal with these above problems: a) use of gonadotropin preparations with reduced LH activity, so-called pure FSH, and b) use of GnRH agonist to suppress endogenous pituitary gonadotropin secretion prior to and during ovarian stimulation.

Characteristics of Different Gonadotropin Preparations

The classical HMG preparation, which has been in clinical use since the beginning of the 1980's, is prepared by extraction from the urine of postmenopausal women, and contains equal activity of FSH and LH. However, in commercial preparations (Humegon, Pergonal) a considerable amount of the LH-like activity derives from HCG, up to 25%[15]. In addition, the specific activity of HMG preparations is low reflected by the fact, that > 95% of the protein content consists of non-specific urinary contaminants[16]. Improved purification procedures allowed for removal of LH from the HMG preparation and was introduced as "pure" FSH (Menogon) in the mid-1980's. This preparation was still a crude urinary extract with a specific activity of FSH similar to that of HMG preparations[16]. Due to the impurities of HMG and "pure" FSH both have to be administered by intramuscular injection. The desirability of more pure FSH preparations led to the development of highly purified urinay FSH (FSH-HP; Metrodin-HP, Serono), which via an immunopurification step attained a purity higher than 95% allowing for s.c. administration[17]. The ultimative purity came with the development of recombinant human FSH (rec.FSH) preparations produced by Chinese Hamster Ovary (CHO) cells, in which the genes encoding the human α and ß FSH subunit have been inserted[18]. Rec.FSH which is close to 100% pure, devoid of non-gonadotropin impurities and without LH activity, has been available for clinical use for the last two years and is administered by s.c. injections. FSH is, whether extracted from urine or produced by CHO cells, heavily glycosylated and has a long terminal half-life of about 9-15 h, which by intramuscular administration may be even longer[19]. Therapeutic levels in the bloodstream may persist for up to 3 days[20].

The half-life of LH is considerably shorter, i.e. about 2 h. After i.m. injection LH levels rise to a maximum of 15% after 2 h, but shortly thereafter, no difference in the concentration of LH can be detected in plasma of women treated with hMG or FSH[21]. Therefore, women treated with exogenous gonadotrophin experience a sustained rise in the concentration of FSH, while the basal concentration of LH (collected at least 18 h after the previous day's injection) usually declines progressively as follicle development occurs[21].

Suppression of Pituitary Gonadotrophin Secretion with GnRH Agonist Combined with Exogenous Gonadotrophins in Ovarian Stimulation

Use of gonadotrophin-releasing hormone agonists (GnRH-a) to suppress the endogenous gonadotropin secretion during ovarian stimulation with exogenous gonadotropins was introduced in the mid-1980's, and proved to be an effective method to prevent an untimely mid-cycle surge of LH and to lower basal secretion of LH during the follicular phase of the cycle[22]. A large meta-analysis of randomized controlled trials showed, that this strategy significantly improved clinical pregnancy rates in IVF compared to other hormone stimulation regimens, however, at the cost of a significantly increased consumption of gonadotropins[23]. While the beneficial effect of a GnRH-a induced elimination of the spontaneous LH surges in IVF treatment cycles is well established, it is not equally well established that the concomitant lowering of basal endogenous LH secretion during the follicular phase also contributes to the increased success rates of IVF treatments. Indeed, it has been proposed that exogenous LH administration for ovarian stimulation may not be required and may even be detrimental to follicle growth and oocyte maturation in normogonadotropic women[6,24]. A number of studies reporting good results by using pure FSH and rec.FSH in combination with GnRH-a down-regulation in IVF support this notion[25,26]. Consequently, replacing HMG, which contains equal amounts of FSH and LH-like activity, with preparations containing only FSH seems a rational approach to ovarian stimulation in IVF cycles. Although this statement might find support in the previously mentioned studies demonstrating a negative impact on oocyte quality, pregnancy rate and incidence of miscarriage by increased serum concentrations of endogenous LH, preferably in women with PCOS[9-12], it is worth mentioning, that no differences in outcome have been demonstrated in studies comparing the effect of ovarian stimulation with FSH and HMG in the treatment of women with PCOS[27].

Conversely, it has actually been suggested that GnRH-a down-regulation in some normogonadotrophic women results in profound suppression of LH levels, that impair oestradiol synthesis due to lack of androgen substrate[28]. Therefore, in cases when "pure" FSH is used for ovarian stimulation in combination with GnRH-a down-regulation, much diminished levels of LH may affect the outcome of IVF negatively. It is therefore possible, that some normogonadotropic women after GnRH-a down-regulation may benefit from HMG instead of FSH preparations devoid of LH activity.

These above arguments pro et contra the use of HMG versus purified FSH (urinary or recombinant) in GnRH-a down-regulated normogonadotrophic women have lead us to ask the following questions:

1. *Is the LH content in HMG preparations detrimental to the outcome of IVF treatment?*
2. *Is there, overall, equality between HMG and purified FSH (urinary or recombinant)?*
3. *Is there a critical lower level of LH and is exogenous LH (HMG or recombinant LH) in some instances needed to improve the outcome of IVF?*

These questions have been addressed in a number of recent studies from our clinic as well as others to be discussed below.

HMG versus Urinary, Highly Purified FSH (FSH-HP)

In a prospective randomized study we compared the effects of hMG and FSH-HP (Metrodin HP, Serono) in 218 normogonadotropic women undergoing IVF treatment[29]. The inclusion criteria were: i) age <40 years; ii) regular menstrual cycle with intervals between 26 and 32 days; iii) pretreatment serum LH and FSH < 10 IU/L, i.e. on cycle day 2 less than 6 months before treatment start; iv) normal semen analysis of the partner at oocyte retrieval. All women were subjected to pituitary down-regulation by a daily subcutaneous injection of 0.5 mg Suprefact (Hoechst, Denmark), starting in the mid-luteal phase, i.e. on cycle day 21. After 14 days, down-regulation was ascertained by vaginal ultrasound examination and serum oestradiol < 200 pmol/L. At this stage the women were randomized to receive either HMG (Personal, Serono Nordic) or FSH-HP (Fertinorm HP = Metrodin-HP, Serono Nordic) in a standardized dose of 225 IU per day for 7 days. Only hereafter could the dosage be individualized according to ovarian response (vaginal ultrasound, serum oestradiol).

In all women blood was sampled routinely firstly on the day when down-regulation was confirmed and gonadotrophin administration started (=stimulation day 1), secondly on stimulation day 8 before gonadotrophin injection was given and 18 hours after the last injection, and finally on the day of oocyte retrieval, i.e 36 h after injection of HCG and about 72 hours after the last

TABLE 1 - *HMG versus FSH-HP. Outcome of stimulation, oocyte retrieval, in-vitro fertilization and pre-embryo development. Values are mean ± SEM per cycle*[29].

	HMG	*FSH-HP*	*P value*
No. of cycles started (%)	114 (100)	104 (100)	
No. of cycles with oocyte retrieval (%)	114 (100)	102 (98)	
No. of cycles with embryo transfer (%)	107 (94)	85 (82)	< 0.05
Duration of stimulation (days)	9.3 ± 0.1	9.3 ± 0.1	
No. of ampoules (75IU) used	28.6 ± 0.1	28.6 ± 0.1	
No. of oocytes retrieved	13.4 ± 0.6	13.7 ± 0.7	
Fertilization rate: %	56	50	< 0.005
No. of transferable embryos	4.0 ± 0.3	3.2 ± 0.4	< 0.01
No. of transferred embryos	1.7 ± 0.1	1.5 ± 0.1	

gonadotrophin injection. The sera were immediately analysed for oestradiol and aliquots frozen and stored for later analysis of FSH and LH.

A total of 114 women were treated with HMG and 104 with FSH-HP. The two groups were comparable with regard to age, duration of infertility, infertility diagnosis and pretreatment basal FSH and LH levels[29].

Table 1. shows, that the number of cycles with oocyte retrieval, mean duration of stimulation (9.3 days), mean number of ampoules used (28.6), number of oocytes retrieved (13.4 versus 13.7) and number of embryos transferred (1.7 versus 1.5) were similar in the hMG and FSH-HP group. By contrast, cancellation of embryo transfer due to complete failure of fertilization was significantly more frequent in the FSH-HP group (18%) than in the hMG group (6%); $p < 0.05$. In addition, fertilization rate and mean number

TABLE 2 - *HMG versus FSH-HP. Serum concentrations of oestradiol, FSH and LH on stimulation day 1 and 8 and on the day of oocyte retrieval 114 women treated with HMG and 104 women treated with FSH-HP. Values are mean±SEM*[29].

	HMG	*FSH-HP*	*P values*
Number of women:	114	104	
Stimulation day 1:			
FSH (IU/L)	3.0 ± 0.1	3.1 ± 0.1	NS
LH (IU/L)	1.7 ± 0.1	1.5 ± 0.1	NS
Oestradiol (pmol/L)	71 ± 2	67 ± 4	NS
Stimulation day 8:			
FSH (IU/L)	11.4 ± 0.3	13.6 ± 0.4	< 0.001
LH (IU/L)	1.2 ± 0.1	0.9 ± 0.1	< 0.02
Oestradiol (pmol/L)	3324 ± 254	2160 ± 229	< 0.01
Day of oocyte retrieval:			
FSH (IU/L)	5.8 ± 0.2	8.0 ± 0.8	< 0.001
LH (IU/L)	0.2 ± 0.02	0.2 ± 0.02	NS

NS = not significant.

of transferable embryos per cycle were significantly higher in the hMG group compared to the FSH-HP group, $p < 0.005$ and < 0.01, respectively (Table 1). No significant differences were observed between the HMG group and the FSH-HP group with regard to delivery rate per started cycle (32% versus 29%), clinical abortion rate (10% versus 14%) or implantation rate (30% versus 30%).

The serum concentration of oestradiol FSH and LH on stimulation day 1 and 8 and on the day of oocyte retrieval are shown in Table 2. On stimulation day 1 these serum hormone concentrations were similar, indicating an equally effective pituitary down-regulation in the two groups of women. On stimulation day 8, however, concentrations of FSH were significantly higher in the FSH-HP group than in the hMG group ($p < 0.001$), in spite of the fact that all women had received the same amount of exogenous FSH, i.e. 21 ampoules of either hMG or FSH-HP. LH levels on stimulation day 8 were lower in both groups than on stimulation day 1, but significantly higher ($p < 0.02$) in the hMG group, who had received exogenous LH (225 IU daily for 7 days), than in the FSH-HP group. In addition, the HMG group showed significantly higher oestradiol levels on stimulation day 8 than did the FSH-HP group ($p < 0.01$).

Is the LH Content in hMG Preparations Detrimental to the Outcome of IVF?

The similar clinical outcome of IVF in GnRH-a down-regulated normogonadotropic women treated with hMG or FSH-HP of the above study, has been confirmed in later studies using similar design[30,31]. Consequently, there is evidence to suggest that the LH levels found in serum of GnRH-a down-regulated women treated with hMG as compared to FSH-HP, do not influence the outcome of IVF treatment negatively.

Is there Equality Between hMG and FSH (Urinary or Recombinant) with Regard to IVF Outcome?

Although the delivery rate per started cycle in the hMG group (32%) and the FSH-HP group (29%) was similar, our results showed important differences between the groups. Thus, the hMG treated patients ran a significantly lower risk of complete failure of fertilization and produced significantly more transferable pre-embryos than those treated with FSH-HP (Table 1). A later Finnish study comparing hMG and FSH-HP in GnRH-a down-regulated fertile oocyte donors confirmed this negative impact of FSH-HP on fertilization rate[30], whereas a study from Britain found similar fertilization rates between hMG and FSH-HP treated patients[31]. By contrast, in a randomized, prospective study comparing the effects of FSH (Metrodin, Serono) and hMG in IVF in 343 women (172 received FSH and 171 received hMG) Daya et al.[32] found a significantly higher proportion of women with complete failure of fertilization in the hMG group compared to the FSH treated women. Although the ongoing pregnancy rate in the FSH group (16.3%) was higher than in the hMG group (9.9%) this difference did not reach statistical significance. Including these results in a meta-analysis of ten other randomized trials of smaller size showing significantly better results with FSH than with hMG, Daya et al. concluded, that the LH activity of hMG was responsible for the poorer results in the hMG treated women[32]. However, a number of differences between our and other studies and that of Daya et al. makes this interpretation controversial. In the meta-analysis, trials with and without GnRH agonist were included. In the study of Daya et al.[32], GnRH-a was used in a flare-up protocol, and down-regulation of LH was assumed but not confirmed by serum LH measurements. In addition, and in contrast to most other studies, serum oestradiol levels were similar in the FSH and hMG group, indicating that differences in LH levels between the two groups of women were small or non-existing, perhaps illustrating that the flare-up protocol results in a less effective reduction of LH levels.

As documented in our study and by others the hormone profiles in GnRH-a down-regulated normogonadotropic women treated with hMG differ significantly from those in women treated with urinary FSH-HP or recombinant, human FSH. Thus, on stimulation day 8 levels of LH and oestradiol were significantly higher in the hMG group than in the FSH-HP group, indicating that the exogenous LH contained in hMG via its stimulation of thecal androgen synthesis contributes to increased oestradiol production in the granulosa layer stimulated by FSH. Therefore, quite surprising was our finding of a significantly higher level of FSH on stimulation day 8 and on the day of oocyte retrieval in the FSH-HP group as compared to the hMG group (Table 2). This discrepancy may be explained by the fact that the distribution of FSH isoforms in FSH-HP (Metrodin-HP, Serono) deviates profoundly of the less purified urinary FSH (Metrodin, Serono), recombinant human FSH (Puregon, Organon) and human pituitary FSH, being far more acidic in nature[33]. Since acidic isoforms have a longer half-life than basic isoforms of FSH, it might be expected that FSH-HP stays longer and accumulates to higher concentrations in serum than do other preparations of FSH.

Could raised levels of FSH then have a negative impact on the outcome of IVF? This question was addressed by us in a retrospective analysis of three groups of pituitary down-regulated normogonadotropic women treated with hMG, FSH-HP or recombinant FSH (Gonal-F, Serono) using a standardized dose of gonadotropins for the first 7 days of stimulation as described above[34]. This analysis showed, as expected, that levels of FSH on stimulation day 8 were significantly higher in the FSH-HP group than in the hMG and rec.FSH groups. Unexpectedly, however, we found a statistically significant negative correlation between FSH levels on stimulation day 8 and oocyte cleavage rate. A ready explanation for this finding is not at hand, but supported by animal studies it is suggested, that supra physiological levels of FSH may induce resumption of oocyte meiosis without inducing the ovulatory process itself, leading to ovulation/retrieval of "aged" oocytes with a reduced potential for fertilization and pre-embryo development[34].

Notwithstanding these theoretical considerations on FSH isoforms, it is well documented in our study as well as in numerous others that the LH content in HMG preparations does make a difference compared to purified FSH preparations, be it FSH-HP or rec.FSH, in relation to oestradiol synthesis during stimulation in pituitary down-regulated, normogonadotropic women. Whether or not this correlates to a negative or positive outcome of IVF treatment is less certain, and will be discussed below.

Is There a Critical Lower Level of LH and is Exogenous LH (hMG or Recombinant LH) in Some Instances Needed to Improve the Outcome of IVF in Normogonadotropic, Pituitary Down-regulated Women?

Administration of rec.FSH to hypogonadotrophic females indicates, that FSH alone can induce follicular growth, whereas oestradiol secretion remains very low. Normal oestradiol secretion requires the presence of LH, as observed when using hMG[35]. It is well known that oestradiol secretion is required for normal endometrial proliferation and, thereby, optimal conditions for implantation in the luteal phase. In addition, it seems that a certain amount of oestradiol in the follicular environment is needed for normal oocyte maturation, fertilsability, and pre-embryo development. Thus, Balasch et al.[36] demonstrated, that oocytes obtained from a hypogonadotropic woman treated with FSH had a reduced fertilisability compared with oocytes from the same woman after treatment with combined FSH and LH (hMG). Further evidence for a specific role of LH activity in securing normal pre-embryo developmental capacity derives from studies in monkeys, in which a profound suppression of pituitary gonadotrophin secretion was effected by treatment with GnRH antagonist of long duration. These monkeys were then treated with recombinant FSH with or without recombinant LH. The study showed, that FSH alone is sufficient for growth of antral follicles and development of meiotically competent oocytes, but exposure to LH or oestradiol improves performance in terms of antral follicular growth, oocyte fertilization and preimplantation embryonic development[5]. Do these findings apply to the situation in the pituitary down-regulated normogonadotropic women, when purified or recombinant FSH is used for ovarian stimulation? Generally, it is believed that in GnRH-a down-regulated normogonadotropic women treated with FSH resting levels of endogenous LH are sufficient for normal follicular development and oocyte maturation. This view is supported by the good results reported on use of rec. FSH in down-regulated women during IVF treatment[26]. However, it may be possible that the serum LH concentration during down-regulation sometimes decline to a level which compromise the ovarian response, and that replacement of FSH with hMG or rec.LH may compensate for this. In a study by Flemming et al.[28] comparing the effects of FSH-HP and hMG in GnRH-a down-regulated women, nearly half of the women (17 of 40) treated with FSH-HP showed consistently low serum LH (< 1 IU/L) and significantly lower serum concentrations of oestradiol. In addition, oestradiol and testosterone concentration in follicular fluid were lower than those found in FSH-HP-treated patients with LH > 1 IU/L and in all patients (N=20) treated with HMG. In a later study from the same group[37] the impact of profound suppression of LH, i.e LH < 0.5 IU/L, in FSH-HP treated patients were investigated. These data showed a significantly lower oestradiol per millimetre total follicular diameter in the group with LH < 0.5 IU/L (N=20) compared to those with LH > 0.5 IU/L (N=41). In the low LH group there was a lower yield of oocytes and lower fertilization rates, although not statistically significant, but a significantly reduced quantity of embryos available for cryopreservation. Supernumerary embryos were cultured for 7 days to determine the blastocyst rate, which was similar in the < 0.5 IU/L and > 0.5IU/L LH groups (27% and 23%, respectively). Thus, there seems to be some effect of a profound suppression of LH in normogonadotropic women, although it apparently did not affect blastocyst development. However, a normal development to the blastocyst stage in vitro does not necessarily imply normal embryonal capacity for implantation and foetal development in vivo.

Indeed, preliminary data from our clinic indicate, that detrimental effects of low LH levels in the follicular phase may become manifest only after implantation. A total of 198 consecutive IVF cycles were analysed retrospectively. The inclusion criteria were i) female age below 40 years, ii) regular menstrual cycles with pretreatment levels of FSH and LH on cycle day 2 below 10 IU/L, iii) standard hormonal treatment as follows: after down-regulation was achieved, all women were treated with recombinant FSH (Gonal-F, Serono) in a standard dose of 225 IU per day for 7 days. Thereafter the dose was individualized according to ovarian response. Blood samples for oestradiol, FSH and LH analysis were obtained on stimulation day 1 and 8.

On stimulation day 8 the concentration of LH in serum was found to be below 0.5 IU/L in 128 of the 198 patients and above 0.5 IU/L in the remaining 70 patients. The outcome of IVF (ICSI included) in the two groups of women with LH below and above 0.5 IU/L is shown in Table 3. As expected, women with LH below the median show serum oestradiol levels significantly lower than those with LH above the median. The mean number of oocytes, fertilization rates and mean number of transferable embryos are similar between the groups. The number of positive pregnancy tests are also similar, but the rate of early pregnancy loss (35%) in the group with LH below 0.5 IU/L is significantly higher than in the group with LH above 0.5 IU/L (8%), $p < 0.05$. The delivery rate per started cycle in the below 0.5 IU/L LH group (19%) is lower than in the above 0.5 IU/L LH group (26%), but not statistically significant, $p > 0.05$.

These preliminary data indicate, that profound suppression of LH in normogonadotropic women treated with rec.FSH devoid of LH activity may have negative effects on the pregnancy outcome. The data also indicate, that a

TABLE 3 - *Outcome of IVF in 198 normogonadotropic, GnRH-a down-regulated, rec.FSH stimulated women related to serum LH concentration below or above 0.5 IU/L on stimulation day 8 (S8).*

	Serum LH concentration on stimulation day 8		
	Se-LH<0.5IU/L	*Se-LH>0.5 IU/L*	*P-value*
No. Cycles	128	70	
Se-E2 (pmol/L) on S8, mean:	1492	3858	< 0.001
No. Oocytes/cycle, mean	12.6	14.6	NS
Rate of fertilized oocytes, mean	63%	64%	NS
Rate of cleaved oocytes, mean	58%	60%	NS
Transferable embryos[1], mean	26%	29%	NS
Positive pregnancy test	31% (40/128)	34% (24/70)	NS
Early pregnancy loss[2]	35% (14/40)	8% (2/24)	< 0.05
Ectopic pregnancy	5% (2/40)	17% (4/24)	NS
Delivery/started cycle	19% (24/128)	26% (18/70)	NS

NS = not significant.
[1] includes the percentage of aspirated oocytes that developed satisfactorily to transfer or cryo-preservation.
[2] includes biochemical pregnancies and clinical spontaneous abortion, but excludes ectopic pregnancies.

substantial number, i.e two thirds, of normogonadotropic women in a standard GnRH-a treatment are suppressed to an extent that is biologically significant. Whether or not these negative effects on pregnancy outcome are mediated by the low oestradiol levels accompanying LH suppression is presently unclear. Also, it is not certain whether administration of exogenous LH as hMG or rec.LH during ovarian stimulation will restore treatment outcome to that seen in women with LH levels above 0.5 IU/L. Only large prospective, randomized trials in down-regulated normogonadotropic women may answer this question. A prospective randomized trial comparing rec.FSH and HMG is now in progress in our clinic.

Conclusions

Available data suggest, that the LH content in hMG preparations do not have a detrimental effect on the outcome of IVF, when compared to use of FSH-HP or rec.FSH for ovarian stimulation in pituitary down-regulated normogonadotropic women. On the contrary, some recent data suggest, that standard pituitary down-regulation with GnRH agonist in a substantial number of normogonadotropic women suppresses endogenous LH secretion to a level at which negative consequences for pregnancy prognosis develop, especially when FSH preparations devoid of LH activity is use for ovarian stimulation. Whether or not addition of LH in the form of rec.LH or hMG will remedy this situation, rely on future prospective, randomized studies comparing the effects of rec.FSH and rec.FSH+rec.LH or HMG with reference to serum LH levels during stimulation.

Acknowledgment

Thanks to Claus Yding Andersen DMSci for intellectual support and fruitful discussions while preparing this manuscript.

References

1. Gore-Langton R.E., Armstrong D.T.: Follicular steroidogenesis and its control. In: Knobil E., Neill J. (eds), *The Physiology of Reproduction.* Raven Press, New York, pp. 571-627, 1994.
2. Yong E.L., Hillier S.G., Turner M., Baird D.T., Ng S.C., Bongso A., Ratnam S.S.: Differential regulation of cholesterol side-chain cleavage (P450scc) and aromatase (P450arom) enzyme mRNA expression by gonadotrophins and cyclic AMP in human granulosa cells. *J. Mol. Endocrinol.*, 12:239-249, 1994.
3. Byskov A.G., Yding Andersen C., Hossaini A., Guoling X.: Cumulus cells of oocyte-cumulus complexes secrete a meiosis activating substance when stimulated with FSH. *Mol. Reprod. Dev.*, 46:296-305, 1997.
4. Tesarik J., Mendoza C.: Non-genomic effects of 17-estradiol on maturing human oocytes: relationship to oocyte developmental potential. *J. Clin. Endocrinol. Metab.*, 80:1438-1443, 1995.
5. Weston A.M., Zelinski-Wooten M.B., Hutchison J.S., Stouffer R.L., Wolf D.P.: Developmental potential of embryos produced by in vitro fertilization from gonadotrophin-releasing hormone antagonist-treated macaques stimulated with recombinant human follicle stimulating hormone alone or in combination with luteinizing hormone. *Hum. Reprod.*, 11:608-613, 1996.
6. Chappel S.C., Howles C.: Reevaluation of the roles of luteinizing hormone and follicle stimulating hormone in the ovulatory process. *Hum. Reprod.*, 6:1206-1212, 1991.
7. Steptoe P.C., Edwards R.G.: Birth after reimplantation of a human embryo [letter]. *Lancet*, ii:336, 1978.
8. Trounson A.O., Leeton J.F., Wood C., Webb J., Wood J.: Pregnancies in human by fertilization in vitro and embryo transfer in the controlled ovu-

latory cycle. *Science,* 212:681-682, 1981.
9. Stanger J.D., Yovich J.L.: Reduced in vitro fertilisation of human oocytes from patients with raised basal luteinizing hormone levels during the follicular phase. *Br. J. Obstet. Gynaecol.*, 92:385-393, 1985.
10. Howles C.M., MacNamee M.C., Edwards R.G., Goswamy R., Steptoe P.C.: Effect of high tonic levels of luteinizing hormone on outcome of in vitro fertilisation. *Lancet,* ii:521-522, 1986.
11. Conway G.S., Honour J.W., Jacobs H.S.: Heterogeneity of the polycystic ovary syndrome: clinical, endocrine and ultrasound features. *Clin. Endocrinol.*, 30:459-470, 1989.
12. Regan L., Owen E.J., Jacobs H.S.: Hypersecretion of luteinizing hormone, infertility and miscarriage. *Lancet,* 336:1141-1144,1989.
13. Shoham Z, Jacobs HS, Insler V. Luteinizing hormone: its role, mechanism of action and detrimental effects when hypersecreted during the follicular phase. *Fertil. Steril.*, 59:1153-1161, 1993.
14. Yding Andersen C.: Characteristics of human follicular fluid associated with successful conception after in vitro fertilization. *J. Clin. Endocrinol. Metab.*, 77:1227-1234, 1993.
15. Stokman P.G.W., Leeuw R., van den Wijngaard H.A.G.W., Kloosterboer H.J., Vemer H.M., Sanders A.L.M.: Human chorionic gonadotrophin in commercial menopausal gonadotropin. *Fertil. Steril.,* 60:175-178, 1993.
16. Giudice E., Crisci C., Eshkol A., Papoian R.: Composition of commercial gonadotrophin preparations extracted from human post-menopausal urine: characterization of non-gonadotrophin proteins. *Hum. Reprod.*, 9:2291-2299, 1994.
17. Le Cotonnec J.-Y., Porchet H.C., Beltrami V.C., Howles C.M.: Comparative pharmacokinetics of two urinary follicle stimulating hormone preparations in healthy female and male volunteers. *Hum. Reprod.*, 8:1604-1611, 1993.
18. Chappel S., Kelton C., Nugent N.: Expression of human gonadotropins by recombinant DNA methods. In: Genazzi A.R., Petraaglia F. (eds), *Proceedings of the 3rd World Congress on Gynecological Endocrinology.* Parthenon Publishing Group, Carnforth, UK, pp. 179-184, 1992.
19. Baird D.T.: In: *Gonadotrophins, Gonadotrphin-releasing Hormone Analogues and Growth Factors in Infertility: Future perspectives.* Howles C.M. (ed). Medifax International, pp. 43-55, 1992.
20. Dicsfalusy E., Harlin J.: Clinical-pharmacological studies on human menopausal gonadotrophin. *Hum. Reprod.*, 3:21-27, 1988.
21. Baird D.T., Howles C.M.: Induction of ovulation with gonadotrophins: HMG versus purified FSH. In: Filicori M., Flamigni C. (eds), *Ovulation*

Induction: Basic Science and Clinical Advances. Elsevier Science BV, Amsterdam, pp. 135-143, 1994.
22. Flemming R., Coutts J.T.R.: Induction of multiple follicular growth in normally menstruating women after gonadotrophin-releasing hormone agonist suppression. *Fertil. Steril.*, 45:226-230, 1986.
23. Hughes E.G., Fedorkow D.M., Daya S., Sagle M.A., Van de Koppel M.B., Collins J.A.: The routine use of gonadotrophin-releasing hormone agonist prior to in vitro fertilization and gamete intrafallopian transfer: a meta-analysis of randomized controlled trials. *Fertil. Steril.*, 58:888-896, 1992.
24. Daya S., Gunby J., Hughes E.G., Collins J.A., Sagle M.A.: Randomized controlled trial of follicle stimulating hormone versus human menopausal gonadotrophin in in-vitro fertilization. *Hum. Reprod.*, 10:392-396, 1995.
25. Edelstein M.C., Brzyski R.G., Jones G.S., Simonetti S., Muasher S.J.: Equivalency of human menopausal gonadotrophin and follicle stimulating hormone stimulation after gonadotrophin-releasing hormone agonist suppression. *Fertil. Steril.*, 53:103-106, 1990.
26. Out H.J., Mannaerts B.M.J.L., Driessen S.G.A.J., Coelingh Bennink H.J.T.: A prospective, randomized, assessor-blind, multicentre study comparing recombinant and urinary follicle-stimulating hormone (Puregon versus Metrodin) in in-vitro fertilization. *Hum. Reprod.*, 10:2534-2540, 1995
27. Homburg R.: Polycystic ovary syndrome - From gynaecological curiosity to multi system endocrinopathy. *Hum. Reprod.*, 11:29-39, 1996.
28. Flemming R., Chung C.C., Yates R.W.S., Coutts J.R.T.: Purified urinary follicle stimulating hormone induces different hormone profiles compared with menotrophins, dependent upon the route of administration and endogenous luteinizing hormone activity. *Hum. Reprod.*, 11:1854-1858.
29. Westergaard L.G., Erb K., Laursen S., Rasmussen P.E., Rex S.: The effect of human menopausal gonadotrophin and highly purified, urine-derived follicle stimulating hormone on the outcome of in-vitro fertilization in down-regulated normogonadotrophic women. *Hum. Reprod.*, 11:1209-1213, 1996.
30. Söderström-Antilla V., Foudila T., Hovatta O.: A randomized comparative study of highly purified FSH and HMG for ovarian hyperstimulation in an oocyte donation programme. *Hum. Reprod.*, 11:1864-1870, 1996.
31. Bagratec J.S., Lockwood G., Lopez Bernal A., Barlow D.H., Ledger W.L.: Comparison of highly purified FSH (Metrodin-High Purity) with Pergonal for IVF superovulation. *J. Ass. Reprod. Gen.*, 15:65-69, 1998.
32. Daya S.: HMG versus FSH: is there a difference? In: Filicori M., Flagmini C. (eds), *Ovulation Induction Update '98.* Proceedings of the 2nd World Conference on Ovulation Induction. The Parthenon Publishing Group,

New York - London, pp. 183-192, 1998.
33. Lambert A., Rodgers M., Mitchell R., Wood A.M., Wardle C., Hilton B., Robertson W.R.: In-vitro biopotency and glycoform distribution of recombinant human follicle stimulating hormone (Org 32489), Metrodin, and Metrodin-HP. *Hum. Reprod.*, 10:1928-1936, 1995.
34. Yding Andersen C., Westergaard L.G., Byskov A.G., Erb K.: Reduced in vitro fertilization of human oocytes correlates with raised circulating FSH levels during ovarian stimulation in normogonadotrophic women down-regulated with GnRH analogues. *J. Ass. Reprod. Gen.*, 14:581-588, 1997.
35. Couzinet B., Lestrat N., Brailly S., Forest M., Schaison G.: Stimulation of ovarian follicular maturation with pure follicle-stimulating hormone in women with gonadotrophin deficiency. *J. Clin. Endocrinol. Metab.*, 66:552-556, 1988.
36. Balasch J., Miro F., Burzaco I., Casamitjana R., Civico S., Ballesca J.L., Puerto B., Vanrell J.A.: The role of luteinizing hormone in human follicle development and oocyte fertility: evidence from in-vitro fertilization in a woman with long-standing hypogonadotrophic hypogonadism and using recombinant human follicle stimulating hormone. *Hum. Reprod.*, 10:1678-1683, 1995.
37. Fleming R., Lloyd F., Herbert M., Fenwick J., Griffiths T., Murdoch A.: Effects of profound suppression of luteinizing hormone during ovarian stimulation on follicular activity, oocyte and embryo function in cycles stimulated with purified follicle stimulating hormone. *Hum. Reprod.*, 13:1788-1792, 1998.

The Role of Luteinizing Hormone
in Folliculogenesis
and Ovulation Induction, pp. 189-199
Editor M. Filicori

Follicular Phase Serum LH Levels and Assisted Reproduction Outcome

R. Fleming

University Department of Obstetrics and Gynaecology
Royal Infirmary, Glasgow (United Kingdom)

Abstract. *The concentration of circulating LH has been shown to influence ovarian follicular responses to FSH through direct effects upon follicular estradiol (E_2) biosynthesis, follicular, and also oocyte developmental capacity.*

The effects of profound suppression of circulating LH during the follicular phase of IVF cycles were explored in normal women during controlled ovarian hyperstimulation (COH) with GnRH-analog and exogenous purified FSH. Total ovarian responses and the capacity of supernumerary embryos to undergo blastocyst formation were examined in groups of patients defined by the concentration of plasma LH in the mid-follicular phase.

A further large scale retrospective evaluation of gross ovarian responses related to mid-follicular LH concentrations was effected in 431 cycles of ovarian stimulation for IVF treated with purified FSH. The group with suppressed LH (<LH) required longer duration of stimulation, a higher proportion of cycles with dose increases, a lower yield of oocytes, and lower number of embryos in cryostorage.

In a prospective study, supernumerary embryos were cultured for 7 days to determine blastocyst development rates, but the degree of LH suppression made no difference to embryo developmental competence as determined by rates of blastocyst formation (nLH, 23%; <LH, 27%).

A retrospective analysis to determine the effects of low follicular phase LH on the cryopreservation programme revealed that the survival rates, embryo development rate, pregnancy and implantation rates were identical in all three groups examined.

In summary, gross ovarian responses were reduced in cycles treated with a GnRH-analog which showed profoundly suppressed LH, although the developmental potential of embryos produced in those cycles was unaffected by the LH status.

Key words. LH, follicle growth, oocyte yield, embryo development, embryo cryopreservation.

Background

Luteinizing hormone (LH) is usually described as one of the two essential gonadotrophins. A trophic hormone in this context implies having the ability to stimulate growth and cellular mitosis, but in fact LH shows no such activity. In terms of follicular growth, LH appears to have more of a permissive or facilitatory function for the principal trophic hormone, FSH and probably other trophic or paracrine factors such as insulin (and/or IGF-1).

As early as 1972[1], it was realised that successful ovulation induction in patients with hypogonadotropic hypogonadism (WHO group 1) required some LH as a component of the exogenous stimulation regimen. Responses of various FSH preparations were compared, with and without different activities of LH added into the stimulation cocktails. It was decided that approximately similar activities of FSH and LH were required for optimal follicular growth, and 75 IU was determined as the best compromise dose unit. These activities were determined by heterologous bioassay systems which had little relevance to the clinical situation, particularly as the clearance rates of FSH and LH are so widely different, with the majority of LH being eliminated within 24h, and FSH being active in the circulation for more than 2 days. Nevertheless, this level of LH was deemed sufficient to support FSH induced follicular growth and estrogen [mainly estradiol, (E_2)] production.

The Functions of LH

There is evidence supporting roles for LH in three particular functions in the life history of ovarian follicles prior to luteinization. The clearest evidence supports a well defined role for LH in steroid biosynthesis, but it also seems to be involved in follicular growth, and maybe also in the development of oocyte competence. It is difficult to determine whether some of these functions are direct or indirect.

Steroid Biosynthesis. The role of LH in steroid biosynthesis, in the follicular phase, is governed by the two cell, two gonadotrophin hypothesis, whereby LH induces androgen biosynthesis in the theca cells, which the FSH stimulated granulosa cells convert to estrogen. This accounts for the appearance of E_2 in the follicular fluid and the peripheral circulation, but an absence of measurable LH leads to negligible E_2 production, even when FSH can stimulate follicular growth[2].

Follicular Growth. It has been proposed that follicular growth in women, at the latter stages of development, may be induced by FSH alone[3]. However, the results of a recent multicentre study with recombinant FSH and recombinant LH treatment of women with hypogonadotropic hypogonadism, suggested that LH actually sensitises follicles to FSH to encourage follicular development as well as hormone secretion[4]. The numbers of follicles developing after a fixed dose of rFSH was much reduced or delayed in the group treated without rLH. The dose of 75 IU rLH per day appeared to be sufficient to facilitate most functions of follicular development.

Oocyte Maturation and Competence. In an *in vitro* small mammal model, Cortvrindt et al.[5] high-lighted the importance of the interaction between LH and the theca cell mass in physiological events as well as follicular endocrinology. Follicles cultured in the presence of rFSH with or without rLH clearly demonstrated a reduced rate of antrum formation, and oocyte nuclear maturation in mouse follicles grown and ovulated in vitro. Of course, these effects may be either direct or indirect.

In a woman with hypogonadotropic hypogonadism undergoing IVF after treatment with purified FSH or FSH with additional E_2, oocytes were obtained which showed poor fertilisation rates. The same individual was subsequently treated with combined FSH and LH (human menopausal gonadotropin; HMG), and the oocytes showed normal fertilization rates, suggesting that the LH depleted environment may yield oocytes with a reduced potential for further development[6].

Further evidence for LH activity during the follicular phase having an impact upon oocyte / embryo competence was provided by studies in macaque monkeys in which the LH was suppressed using a gonadotropin-releasing hormone antagonist, and follicular growth stimulated with rFSH or rFSH with rLH. The experiment showed a confusing combination of results, but reasonable follicular growth and oocyte yields were obtained after stimulation with recFSH alone. However, there was a higher fertilization rate when recFSH was used, compared with a combination of recFSH and recLH [7]. The absence of recLH had a detrimental effect upon embryo cryo-survival, development and implantation after cryopreservation and thawing[8]. These data imply that there may be an undefined physiological role of LH with implications or oocyte maturation and embryo developmental potential.

Conflicts of Clinical Observations

In the clinical situation of assisted reproduction, the two most important criteria are numbers of oocytes obtained after a course of stimulation, and their developmental competence.

It is clear that the widespread use of urinary FSH or purified urinary FSH, without LH supplementation in COS, has not led to a drop in overall programme success rates, and a number of reports have suggested that there is no need to explore the requirement for LH supplementation further[9]. The introduction of rFSH, which has different isoform profiles from urinary derived FSH and is probably, thereby, more potent[10] appears to show increased efficacy and improved pregnancy rates by comparison with purified FSH treatment[11]. The control experiment comparing rFSH with HMG as ovarian stimulant has not been carried out.

However, different hormone profiles have been recorded when even relatively mild GnRH-a regimens have been used[12,13], and the exploration of other possible effects of LH depletion after GnRH-a co-treatment have been rare.

Loumaye et al.[3] were unable to determine any effects of suppressed LH in COS in normal women treated with FSH, in combined data from their studies, where they assessed LH at the start of treatment and at the time of HCG administration. They did observe a very low pregnancy rate in a group of women with a low E2 concentration (at HCG administration) per oocyte obtained, which is at least a theoretical consequence of LH depletion, although no such relationship was determined.

Estimations of LH Activity

It is difficult to effect reliable and precise LH measurements at the low concentrations in serum experienced during COS, and 24h urinary output also has intrinsic limitations. The concentrations of LH may fluctuate through the 24h between single blood sample analyses, particularly when intranasal spray administration is used. Depo preparations are likely to be more consistent in this respect.

Commercial assays for LH often claim similar low sensitivities and high precision rates, but they clearly do not show the same characteristics at these low concentrations. Figure 1 shows the distribution of LH concentrations values obtained in the mid-follicular phase of COS cycles in 2 different assays. The assay showing >40% of values <0.5IU/L would be clearly inappropriate to explore the effects of LH suppression in a proportion of the population that may be most affected by the phenomenon. When the other assay (D) was used, a statistically normal distribution of concentrations was observed within the 'measurable' range: above 0.5 IU/L. Using this assay to discriminate between the LH values, the endocrine effects of suppressed LH were clearly demonstrated in the follicular fluids (Table 1) and the peripheral circulation (Figure 2) of women undergoing COS for IVF when treated with purified FSH (Metrodin-HP, Serono Laboratories UK; MHP). The women in whom the LH

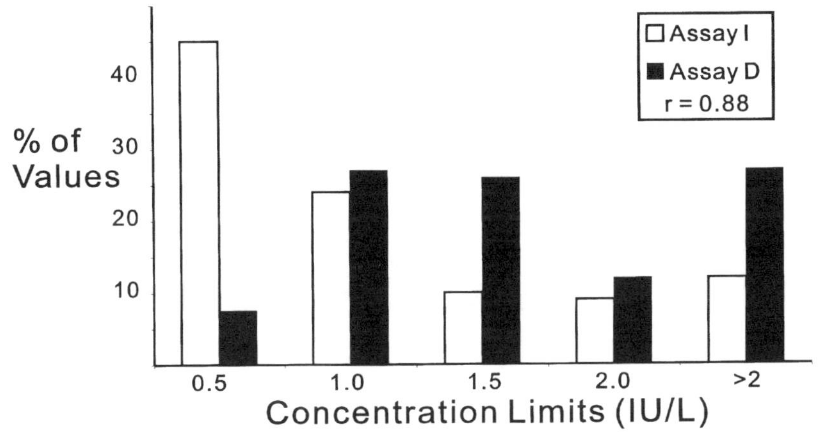

FIGURE 1 - *LH concentrations in mid-follicular phase samples of women undergoing COS determined by 2 different commercial immunoassays.*

was suppressed below 1 IU/L (MHP<LH) showed significantly reduced E_2 secretion throughout the first week of stimulation compared with the group with LH > 1 and also the group treated with hMG.

It is important to note that the concentration of LH at the start of stimulation in COS, although low, is significantly higher than that seen during treatment[14] and the correlation between the values is not strong (r=0.6). This implies that there may be a combined effect of the GnRH-A treatment and a negative feedback action controlling the output of immunoassayable LH.

TABLE 1 - *Concentrations of steroids in the follicular fluids of patients at IVF after COS with either HMG or purified FSH. The latter group was split into sub-groups with either profoundly suppressed mid-follicular LH (MHP<LH) or normal range (MHPnLH) LH concentrations.*

	HMG Mean (s.d.)	*MHP<LH* Mean (s.d.)	*MHP>LH* Mean (s.d.)
n	15	13	21
E2 (ng/ml)	864 (318)	410 (236)*	663 (361)
T (ng/ml)	9.53 (2.51)	6.20 (1.47)*	7.92 (2.66)
P (ng/ml)	15600 (3720)	17192 (3521)	16578 (3823)

*p<0.05 comparing MHP<LH with either of the other 2 groups.

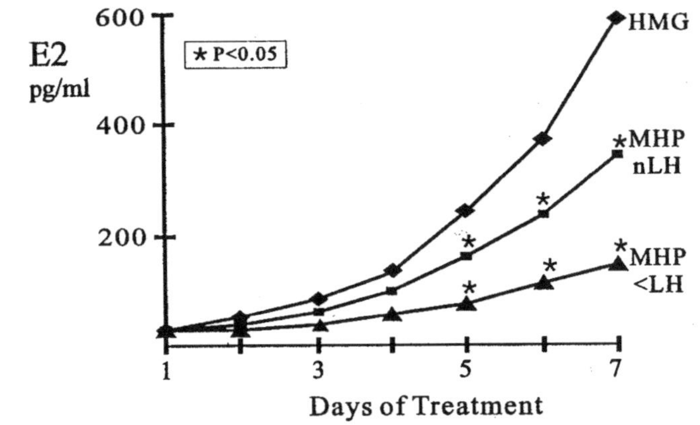

FIGURE 2 - *E_2 responses of patients undergoing COS where the stimulant is either HMG or purified FSH. The cases of purified FSH are separated into those with suppressed LH (MHP<LH) or normal LH (MHPnLH, > 1.0 IU/L).*

When depo GnRH-a formulations are used the LH is consistently lower than with the intranasal spray, but other changes may be beyond the detectable limits of the assays. Mean values from a comparative randomised study where

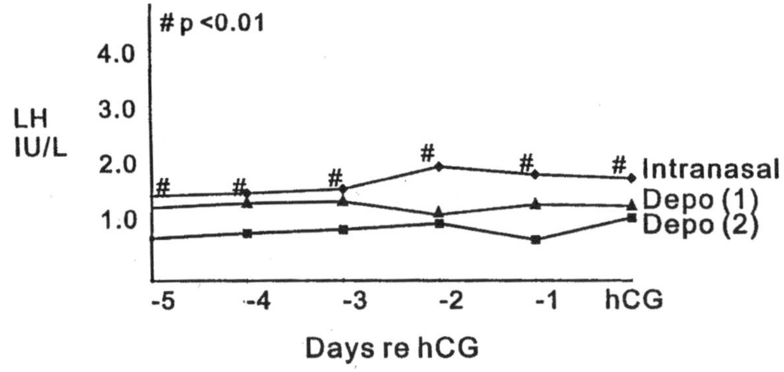

FIGURE 3 - *Late follicular phase LH concentrations in COS cycles where the GnRH-a is given by intra-nasal spray or depo formulations. The 2 depo groups represent mean concentrations seen when the stimulation was initiated soon after menses (Depo1) or following a delay of >9 days (Depo 2).*

the samples were assayed in a batch to avoid interassay variation, are shown in Figure 3.

Figure 2 and table 1 show that reduced E_2 secretion and follicular fluid testosterone values were observed when the mid-follicular phase LH was profoundly suppressed in women treated with COS using purified FSH. The data are clear and they indicate that other possible sequelae of this real effect should be explored on greater depth.

Retrospective Analyses of the Treatment Database

Following the above observations and additional investigations suggesting that there may be a reduced degree of follicular development in the cases with suppressed LH, we carried out a review of the whole treatment database of patients treated with purified FSH. We wished to determine if increasing the numbers may render the observation more secure in mathematical significance. We retrospectively analysed the LH value on stimulation days 6 and 7 for all COS cycles on the database treated with purified FSH (Metrodin-HP; MHP; n = 430), and defined the cases with mid-follicular phase LH concentrations <1.0 IU/L (MHP<LH), and those above (MHPnLH).

Figure 4 shows the differences in treatment duration, oocyte yields, embryo yields and cases with sufficient good quality embryos to qualify for the cryopreservation programme. All parameters were significantly different (P<0.005)

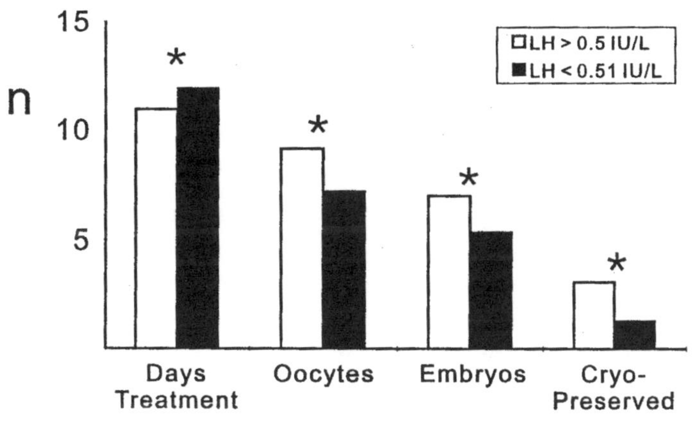

FIGURE 4 - *Impact of suppressed follicular phase LH upon responses to COS with purified FSH (n=430 cycles). *All points significant at p<0.005.*

showing that the MHP<LH group performed less well throughout the programme, in terms of gross ovarian responses. The combined observation of a longer treatment duration with a reduced oocyte yield obviates the criticism that the HCG administration was prejudiced by the E_2 profiles, and it also indicates the important effect of suppressed follicular phase LH. There appeared to be no difference in fertilization rates, or pregnancy rates per transfer.

The effect of a reduced yield of oocytes was reflected in the lower proportion of cycles in the MHP<LH group with embryo cryopreservation and in the pregnancy rates within the cryopreservation programme. The MHP<LH group showed a lower proportion of patients with cryostorage, a lower number of embryo thaws ($p<0.001$) and a lower pregnancy rate ($P<0.05$).

In order to test the observation in a more homogeneous group of unselected patients we effected similar analyses in cases which were the patient's first treatment cycle only within the same database (n=154). All patients started with a fixed dose of 225IU MHP per day. Similar observations were recorded to those in the whole database. Furthermore, the frequency of dose increases at the first monitoring assessment point (stimulation day 7) was highly significantly associated with MHP<LH group ($P<0.0004$). The criteria for dose increases at S7 were ultrasound evidence of insufficient follicular development, with the insurance that the E_2 value did not indicate the presence of more follicles than were observed. In fact, nearly all the cases with dose increases fell within the MHP<LH group.

There are important cost implications of these observations, since this group also showed a longer treatment duration and a lower yield of oocytes.

The Impact of Suppressed Follicular Phase LH upon Developmental Potential of Cryopreserved Embryos

The observation of a lower pregnancy rate of patients with suppressed LH in the cryopreservation programme appeared to relate mainly to a reduced number of embryos available. However, evidence from primate studies indicated that stimulation with rFSH and rLH yield embryos with greater implantation potential after freezing and thawing than did stimulation with rFSH alone.

We investigated this phenomenon in the extended database described above, and Figure 5 shows the results of 3 groups analysed. Patients treated with HMG (n=159), MHPnLH (n=48) and MHP<LH (n=27) yielded embryos with similar thaw survival rates, and in vitro development rates. There were virtually identical rates of pregnancy and embryo implantation observed amongst all 3 groups.

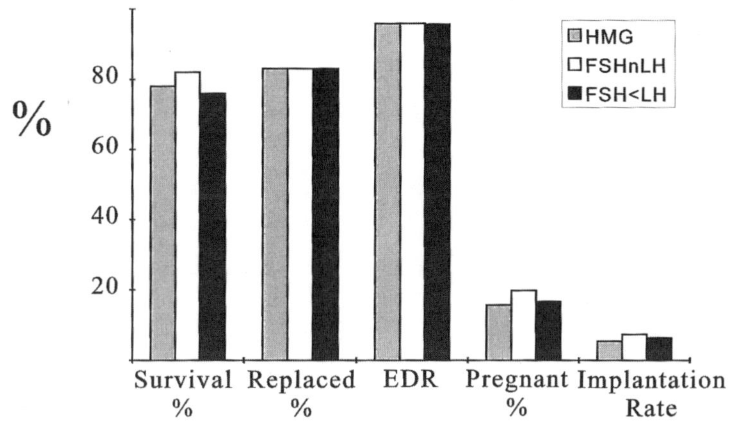

FIGURE 5 - *The impact of suppressed follicular phase LH upon the principal parameters of the cryoembryology programme. The embryo development rate (EDR) is the laboratory assessment of division and conformity of the embryos by reference to standard rates presented as a percentage.*

The Impact of Suppressed Follicular Phase LH upon Blastocyst Development *in vitro*

The effects of profound suppression of circulating LH during the follicular phase of IVF cycles were explored in normal women undergoing COS with GnRH-a and purified FSH. The capacity of supernumerary embryos to undergo blastocyst formation were examined daily in groups of patients defined by the concentration of plasma LH in the mid-follicular phase. LH concentrations <0.5 IU/L diagnosed the group with profoundly suppressed LH (MHP<LH, n=20), which was compared with the remaining patients (MHPn-LH, n=41). As before, the MHP<LH group showed lower estradiol (E_2) concentrations through stimulation. The combined effects of a trend to lower yield of oocytes (not significant) and a lower fertilisation rate (not significant) resulted in a significantly reduced quantity of embryos available for incubation or cryopreservation after the fresh transfer.

All supernumerary embryos were cultured for 7 days to determine blastocyst development rates, and the speed at which the blastocysts were formed. The degree of LH suppression made no difference to either marker of embryo developmental competence, as by day 7 the MHPnLH group showed 23% of embryos had formed blastocysts, while the figure was 27% of embryos in the MHP<LH group. Furthermore, there was no difference in the timing of blastocyst formation between the groups.

It is possible that in the future, improved culture conditions for blastocyst development may allow a more sensitive investigation of the effects of profound LH suppression, but there is no indication of such an effect under these conditions.

Conclusions

The combined effect of these prospective and retrospective studies, is to demonstrate and confirm that the circulating LH in the follicular phase of COS cycles for IVF is important for gross ovarian responses. The principal effect appears to be that low LH activity is associated with reduced gross ovarian responses in the form of follicular development, as well as E_2 secretion.

The reduced yield of oocytes in the LH suppressed group resulted in a lower pregnancy rate within the cryopreservation programme. However, none of the tests of embryo viability - *in vitro* culture of fresh or cryopreserved embryos, or the *in vivo* capacity for implantation appeared to be influenced by the degree of LH suppression.

References

1. Bertrand P.V., Coleman J.R., Crooke A.C., Macnaughton M.C., Mills I.H.: Human ovarian response to gonadotrophins with different ratios of folicle stimulating hormone: luteinizing hormone assessed by different parameters. *J. Endocrinol.*, 53:231-248, 1972
2. Couzinet B., Lestrat N., Brailly S., Forest M., Schaison G.: Stimulation of ovarian follicular maturation with pure follicle stimulating hormone in women with gonadotropin deficiency. *J. Clin. Endocrinol. Metab.*, 66:552-556, 1988.
3. Loumaye E., Engrand P., Howles C.M., O'Dea L.: Assessment of the role of serum luteinizing hormone and estradiol response to follicle stimulating hormone on invitro fertilization treatment outcome. *Fertil. Steril.*, 67:889-899, 1997.
4. The European Recombinant Human LH Study Group: Recombinant Human Luteinizing Hormone (LH) to Support Recombinant Human Follicular Stimulating Hormone (FSH)-Induced Follicular Development in LH- and FSH- deficient anovulatory Women: A Dose Finding Study. *J. Clin. Endocrinol. Metab.*, 83:1507-1514, 1998.
5. Cortvrindt R., Hu Y., Smitz J.: Recombinant luteinizing hormone as a

survival and differentiation factor increases oocyte maturation in recombinant follicle stimulating hormone-supplemented mouse pre-antral follicle culture. *Hum. Reprod.*, 14:1292, 1998.
6. Balasch J., Miro F., Burzaco I., Casamitjana R., Civico S., Ballesca J.L., Puerto B., Vanrell J.A.: The role of luteinizing hormone in human follicle development and oocyte fertility: evidence from in-vitro fertilization in a woman with long-standing hypogonadotrophic hypogonadism and using recombinant human FSH. *Hum. Reprod.*, 10:1678-1683, 1995.
7. Zelinski-wooten M.B., Hutchison J.S., Hess D.L., Wolf D.P., Stouffer R.L.: Follicle stimulating hormone alone supports follicle growth and oocyte development in gonadotrophin-releasing hormone antagonist-treated monkeys. *Human Reprod.*, 10:1658-1666, 1996.
8. Weston A.M., Zelinsky Wooten M.B., Hutchison J.S.: Developmental potential of embryos produced by in-vitro fertilization from gonadotrophin releasing hormone antagonist treated macaques stimulated with recombinant human follicle stimulating hormone in combination with LH. *Hum. Reprod.*, 11:608-613, 1996.
9. Hull M.G.R., Armatage R.J., McDermott A.: Use of follicle stimulating hormone alone (urofollitropin) to stimulate the ovaries for assisted conception after pituitary desensitization. *Fertil. Steril.*, 62:997-1003, 1994.
10. De Leeuw R., Mulders J., Voortman G., Rombout F., Damm J., Klosterboer L.: Structure-function relationship of recombinant follicle stimulating hormone (Puregon). *Hum. Reprod.*, 2:361-369, 1996.
11. Out HJ, Mannaerts BMJ, Drieeson SGAJ, and Coelingh Bennink HJT.: A prospective randomized, assessor-blind, multicentre study comparing recombinant and urinary follicle stimulating hormone (Puregon versus Metrodin) in in-vitro fertilization. *Hum. Reprod.*, 10, 2534-2540, 1995.
12. Fried G., Harlin J., Csemiczky G., Wramsby H.: Controlled ovarian stimulation using highly purified FSH results in a lower serum oestradiol profile in the follicular phase as compared with hMG. *Hum. Reprod.*, 11:474-477, 1996.
13. Fleming R., Chung C.C., Yates R.W.S., Coutts J.R.T.: Purified urinary follicle stimulating hormone induces different hormone profiles compared with menotrophins, dependent upon route of administration and endogenous luteinizing hormone activity. *Hum Reprod.*, 11:1854-1858, 1996
14. Fleming R., Lloyd F., Herbert M., Fenwick J., Griffiths T., Murdoch A.: Effect of profound suppression of luteinizing hormone during ovarian stimulation on follicular activity, oocyte and embryo function in cycles stimulated with purified follicle stimulating hormone. *Hum. Reprod.*, 13:1788-1792, 1998.

The Role of Luteinizing Hormone
in Folliculogenesis
and Ovulation Induction, pp. 201-210
Editor M. Filicori

Effects of Menotropin Luteinising Hormone Content on Oocyte and Embryo Quality

U.D. Gordon

Center for Reproductive Medicine, University of Bristol, Bristol (United Kingdom)

Abstract. *It is now well accepted that follicle stimulating hormone (FSH) alone can induce follicular growth and development but a small amount of luteinising hormone (LH) is necessary for adequate steroidogenesis. However, the effect of menotropin LH content on oocyte maturation, fertilisation and embryo development is less well defined.*

With the advent of purified urinary FSH preparations and more recently recombinant gonadotropins, animal and human studies have confirmed the synergistic role of LH in promoting FSH induced follicular growth. Presence of LH allows for the development of a more optimal cohort of follicles and oestradiol (E_2) secretion. While oocyte nuclear maturity appears independent of follicular phase LH concentrations, the fertilisation potential of the oocyte appears to be compromised in a reduced LH environment.

In contrast to non-human primate work, human embryo cryosurvival and percentage blastocyst development appear not to be affected. However, the number of embryos available may be reduced with low LH due to lower fertilisation rates. In addition, preparations devoid of LH have to-date not resulted in a pregnancy in hypogonadotropic women demonstrating the significance of LH in implantation.

While the mechanism by which LH exerts it's role may be mediated through it's effect on steroidogenesis, further work is required to clarify the precise mechanism of action, optimal dosage and timing of administration.

Key words. Luteinising hormone, follicle stimulating hormone, oocyte fertilisation, embryo development.

Introduction

It is becoming increasingly apparent that hormonal events before the mid-cycle LH peak, specifically the levels of LH and FSH during the early follicular phase, may significantly influence the developmental capacity of the oocyte.

The growth phase of the oocyte is a period of intense metabolic activity and many of the proteins and much of the RNA required during the early embryonic cleavage stages are thought to be generated in the oocyte both before and following the initiation of meiosis[1].

Earlier studies have shown a detrimental effect of high levels of LH in the follicular phase on oocyte maturation, fertilization and conception[2-4]. However, these studies were referring to concentrations of LH >10 IU/L. With the advent of gonadotropin releasing hormone analogues (GnRH-a), pituitary suppression is now routine in most clinics and those high levels of LH are unlikely to be achieved.

Follicle stimulating hormone monotherapy has also come into increasing use based on the perception that LH is needed in only very small amounts during the follicular phase. Studies in women undergoing in vitro fertilisation (IVF) with GnRH-a and purified urinary FSH (uFSH) treatment have shown ovarian responses similar to that of human menopausal gonadotropin (hMG)[5,6]. However, an effect of LH cannot be excluded in these studies as uFSH preparations contain a small amount of LH[7], and even following prolonged pituitary down-regulation there is still endogenous LH present[8]. With the availability of recombinant gonadotropins[9], it is now possible to revisit and study the precise roles of FSH and LH in follicular/oocyte growth and development.

Studies in hypogonadotropic hypogonadal women using recombinant FSH (rhFSH) have confirmed that follicular development can proceed in the presence of FSH alone, however, a small amount of LH is necessary for adequate steroidogenesis[10-12]. What is yet to be ascertained, however, is the role of LH in oocyte maturation, fertilisation and embryo development.

Influence on the follicular phase

Studies in both human and non-human primates have shown that the follicular developmental potential is influenced by LH. The presence of LH appears to facilitate a shortening of the follicular phase and/or a reduction in the amount of gonadotropin ampoules required. Zelinski-Wooten et al.[13] treated macaques with GnRH-antagonist Antide for a period of 90 days to achieve suppression of endogenous LH comparable to hypophysectomised animals. They showed that an average of 12 days was needed to achieve follicular growth with rhFSH compared to 9 days with rhFSH plus recombinant LH (rhLH) treatment. No difference was noted in the number of follicles recruited or the oocytes collected. Shoham et al.[14] compared hMG treatment with uFSH in subsequent cycles in patients with isolated hypogonadotropic hypogonadism and found that the former required significantly fewer number of ampoules of gonadotropin. Balasch et al.[15] compared rhFSH, hMG and uFSH plus oestradiol valerate in a patient with isolated congenital gonadotropin deficiency and showed that the number of gonadotropin ampoules used was lower in the hMG cycle.

It can be speculated that the shorter interval of follicular growth in the presence of LH may influence the quality of the oocyte ultimately affecting the fertilisation/embryo development potential. Studies in immature female rats rendered hypogonadotropic by hypophysectomy[16] or luteinising hormone releasing hormone-antagonist[17] have also shown that while FSH alone can induce multiple follicular development, the addition of a small amount of human chorionic gonadotropin (hCG) increased the percentage of healthy follicles and reduction in atresia in various follicle size classes. The European Recombinant Human LH Study Group[18] investigated the efficacy of rhLH for supporting rhFSH induced follicular development in hypogonadotropic hypogonadal women. Supplementation with 75 IU rhLH resulted in optimal follicular development and luteinisation in the majority of patients.

Oocyte maturity

Maturity of the oocyte is a complex issue and the majority of studies use morphological parameters for assessment, which are subjective. Imthurn et al.[19] used cumulus denuded oocytes for intracytoplasmic sperm injection treatment and found a significantly higher proportion of metaphase-II oocytes with uFSH than hMG treatment (88.8% vs. 80.6%). A higher proportion of oocytes with dark cytoplasm were noted with the hMG group. However, one major limitation of this study was that the clinician taking decisions about the timing of administration of hCG was not blind to the stimulation regime. Mercan et al.[20] compared uFSH treatment with combined FSH/hMG in patients undergoing IVF, and concluded that the percentage of mature oocytes with 'typical desired morphology' was significantly higher with FSH-only group. However, the study was retrospective, with the stimulation protocol based on patient's prior IVF experience, and no difference was noted in the overall percentage of mature oocytes and fertilisation rates.

In contrast, Tornell et al.[21] showed that while both rhFSH and rhLH were independently capable of causing germinal vesicle breakdown in isolated preovulatory rat follicles, a combination of these gonadotropins in submaximal concentrations resulted in an additive effect on oocyte meiosis. In a randomised prospective study in GnRH-a suppressed IVF patients, we compared rhFSH treatment with urinary gonadotropin preparations containing 1, 25 and 75 IU of LH per ampoule, keeping the FSH dose constant[22]. A lower percentage of mature oocytes and a higher percentage of immature oocytes were noted with rhFSH treatment compared to the other three groups. However, the percentage difference (median 96% rhFSH vs 100% other groups), in real terms, was small and not clinically significant.

Fertilisation

While studies in monkeys have shown significantly higher fertilisation rates with rhFSH treatment compared to rhFSH plus rhLH (mean 89% vs 52% respectively), this is in contrast to work published from human studies. Westergaard et al.[23] showed the mean fertilisation rate to be significantly higher with hMG (56%) compared to uFSH (50%) in their randomised trial of down-regulated normogonadotropic women. Soderstrom-Antilla et al.[24] compared uFSH with hMG in their oocyte donation programme and showed higher fertilisation with hMG (36% vs 48% respectively). In a woman with isolated congenital gonadotropin deficiency, oocytes obtained in a LH depleted environment showed considerably lower fertilisation rates with rhFSH or uFSH (27-28%) than with hMG (93%)[15].

Fleming et al.[25] have identified a subgroup of patients on GnRH-a and purified uFSH treatment who show profound suppression of endogenous LH. These cases, with mean serum follicular phase LH levels ≤ 0.5 IU/L, showed significantly lower E_2 levels in the circulation and lower oocyte fertilisation rates[26]. Concern has also been raised about a higher incidence of failed fertilisation in IVF cycles with low LH. Westergaard et al.[23], in their randomised trial comparing uFSH with hMG, reported a significantly higher percentage of complete failure of fertilisation with uFSH (16% vs 6% respectively). In our randomised prospective study on GnRH-a suppressed IVF patients, we reported a dose-related increase in the incidence of complete fertilisation failure with decreasing exogenous LH (17.6%, 13%, 11% and 0% for rhFSH, Metrodin, Normegon and Humegon respectively)[22]. Whether this is related to a more profound suppression of endogenous LH in these specific cases is presently being evaluated.

In contrast, Daya et al.[27] compared uFSH treatment with hMG, and showed a higher number of failed fertilisation cycles with hMG (8% vs 17%, p = 0.047). However, the study included male factor patients and short protocol regimen for pituitary desensitisation with the known 'flare-up' effect, both of which could have influenced the results[28].

Cleavage

Results with regard to the role of LH in embryo development vary. A few clinical studies examined the effects of different urinary gonadotropin preparations on embryo cleavage rates following IVF, and reported no significant differences[5,29-31]. In contrast, others reported better cleavage rates[24] and more transferable embryos[23] with hMG treatment compared to uFSH. Embryo viability and pre-implantation development were also shown to be optimal in GnRH-antagonist treated macaques when folliculogenesis occurred in the presence of exogenous LH[32]. A significant difference in embryo cryosurvival (56% after rhFSH vs 78% after rhFSH + rhLH) and developmental rate to the hatched blastocyst stage (12 days vs 10 days respectively) was noted. The rescue of the corpus luteum also occurred later (16 days vs 12-13 days respectively). Based on these findings, Rekha et al.[33] carried out a retrospective analysis to determine whether follicular phase LH concentration low enough to influence E_2 biosynthesis also influenced cryopreserved embryo development in human IVF cycles.

They found that the embryo survival, development, implantation and pregnancy rates were similar irrespective of the LH concentration recorded in the mid-follicular phase. Fleming et al.[26] showed that while the degree of LH suppression in the follicular phase influenced the number of embryos available, due to a lower oocyte yield and fertilisation rates, no impact was noted upon the fertilised embryos to undergo cleavage and expanded blastocyst formation.

Implantation

Rekha et al.[33] showed no correlation of circulating LH to implantation and pregnancy rates in GnRH-a suppressed IVF patients. In contrast, Weston et al.[32] showed that embryos derived from rhFSH alone without any added LH undergo delayed development in vitro leading to a decreased frequency of implantation in macaques. While 2 pregnancies resulted from three embryo transfer attempts with rhFSH plus rhLH treatment, one twin pregnancy resulted from 8 embryo transfer attempts in the rhFSH only group. Unpublished data from our randomised study also showed significantly different implantation rates with varying amounts of LH. An increasing trend was noted with increasing LH dose (19%, 10%, 18% and 28% for rhFSH, Metrodin, Normegon and Humegon respectively (34). In addition, while pregnancies have been reported in hypogonadal women treated with rhFSH and rhLH[35,36], no pregnancies to date have been documented with rhFSH alone.

Mechanism of LH Action

The precise mechanism of action is yet to be understood. Whether the aforementioned effects of LH are mediated through a more optimal E_2 micro-environment or through a direct action of LH needs to be ascertained. Using 3ß-hydroxysteroid dehydrogenase inhibitor trilostane, follicular growth and oocyte meiotic competence have been shown to be independent of E_2 concentrations in non-human primates[37]. However, significantly lower fertilisation rate was noted with the trilostane treated group compared to the controls. Fleming et al.[26] also showed lower fertilisation rates in the subgroup of patients with very low LH/E_2 concentrations. A direct role for LH, however, cannot be excluded as supplementation of uFSH with oestradiol valerate did not improve the fertilisation rates in a woman with congenital gonadotropin deficiency[15].

One explanation for the better implantation rates noted in the presence of LH could be related to better functional maturity of the oocytes leading to improved oocyte and embryo performance. A second explanation could be related to the differences in the steroidogenic response on endometrial development and a third explanation may be a direct effect of LH on the endometrium. Binding sites for hCG/LH have been identified by immunohistochemistry in both the glandular and the stromal component of the endometrium (38). However, Li et al.[39], in their retrospective study, correlated the follicular phase LH concentrations with endometrial biopsies obtained in the luteal phase. No relationship was noted in the follicular LH concentrations and endometrial development in the peri-implantation period.

Conclusions

Follicular growth can take place in the presence of FSH alone, however LH appears to have a synergistic action in facilitating the rate of growth and development of a more optimal cohort of follicles. Oocyte meiosis appears to be independent of the follicular phase levels of LH/E_2 in non-human primates but data are as yet inconclusive in the human. Oocyte fertilisation potential, however, seems to be compromised by low follicular phase LH. While this may be related to a reduction in the steroid milieu secondary to low LH concentrations, a direct effect of LH on cytoplasmic/membrane events in oocyte maturation cannot be excluded. In variance to non-human primate studies, LH suppression appears to have no impact on embryo cryosurvival and percentage development to the blastocyst stage. However, the number of embryos available may be reduced with low LH due to lower fertilisation rates. Data relating to implantation potential is sparse and further work is awaited.

References

1. Motlik J., Kopency V., Pivko J., Fulka J.: Distribution of proteins labelled during meiotic maturation in rabbit and pig eggs at fertilisation. *J. Reprod. Fertil.*, 58:415-419, 1980.
2. Stanger J.D., Yovich J.L.: Reduced in-vitro fertilisation of human oocytes from patients with raised basal luteinising hormone levels during the follicular phase. *Br. J. Obstet Gynaecol.*, 92:385-393, 1985.
3. Homburg R., Armar N.A., Eshel A., Adams J., Jacobs H.S.: Influence of serum luteinising hormone concentrations on ovulation, conception, and early pregnancy loss in polycystic ovary syndrome. *Br. Med. J.*, 297:1024-1026, 1988.
4. Regan L., Owen E.J., Jacobs H.S.: Hypersecretion of luteinising hormone, infertility, and miscarriage. *Lancet*, 336:1141-1144, 1990.
5. Bentick B., Shaw R.W., Iffland C.A., Burford G., Bernard A.: A randomised comparative study of purified follicle stimulating hormone and human menopausal gonadotropin after pituitary desensitisation with buserelin for superovulation and in vitro fertilisation. *Fertil. Steril.*, 50:79-84, 1988.
6. Hull M.G.R., Armatage R.J., McDermott A.: Use of follicle stimulating hormone alone (urofollitropin) to stimulate the ovaries for assisted conception after pituitary desensitisation. *Fertil. Steril.*, 62:997-1003, 1994.
7. Giudice E., Crisci C., Eshkol A., Papoian R.: Composition of commercial gonadotropin preparations extracted from human post-menopausal urine: characterisation of non-gonadotropin proteins. *Hum. Reprod.*, 9:2291-2299, 1994.
8. Cedars M.I., Lapolt P., Surrey E., Meldrum D.R., Hamilton F.: Leuprolide acetate lowers circulating bioactive luteinising hormone and testosterone concentrations during ovarian stimulation for oocyte retrieval. *Fertil. Steril.*, 53:627-631, 1990.
9. Keene J.L., Matzuk M.M., Otani T., Fauser B.C., Galway A.B., Hsueh A.J., Boime I.: Expression of biologically active human follitropin in Chinese hamster ovary cells. *J. Biol. Chem.*, 246:4769-4775, 1989.
10. Schoot D.C., Coelingh Bennink H.J.T., Mannaerts B.M.L.J., Lamberts S.W.J., Bouchart P., Fauser B.C.J.M.: Human recombinant follicle stimulating hormone induces growth of preovulatory follicles without concomitant increase in androgen and oestrogen biosynthesis in a woman with isolated gonadotropin deficiency. *J. Clin. Endocrinol. Metab.*, 74:1471-1473, 1992.
11. Schoot D.C., Harlin J., Shoham Z., Mannaerts B.M.L.J., Lahlou N., Bouchart P., Coelingh Bennink H.J.T., Fauser B.C.J.M.: Recombinant human follicle stimulating hormone and ovarian response in gonadotropin defi-

cient women. *Hum. Reprod.*, 9:1237-1242, 1994.
12. Shoham Z., Mannaerts B., Insler V., Coelingh-Bennick H.: Induction of follicular growth using recombinant human follicle stimulating hormone in two volunteer women with hypogonadotropic hypogonadism. *Fertil. Steril.*, 59:738-742, 1993.
13. Zelinski-Wooten M.B., Hutchison J.S., Hess D.L., Stouffer R.L.: Follicle stimulating hormone alone supports follicle growth and oocyte development in gonadotropin-releasing hormone antagonist-treated monkeys. *Hum. Reprod.*, 10(7):1658-1666, 1995.
14. Shoham Z., Balen A., Patel A., Jacobs H.S.: Results of ovulation induction using human menopausal gonadotropins or purified follicle-stimulating hormone in hypogonadotropic hypogonadism patients. *Fertil. Steril.*, 56: 1048-1053, 1991.
15. Balasch J., Miro F., Burzaco I., Casamitjama R., Scivico S., Ballesca J.L., Puerto B., Vanrell J.A.: The role of luteinising hormone in human follicle development and oocyte fertility: evidence from in-vitro fertilisation in a woman with long-standing hypogonadotropic hypogonadism and using recombinant human follicle stimulating hormone. *Hum. Reprod.*, 10(7): 1678-1683, 1995.
16. Mannaerts B., Uilenbroek J., Schoot P., de Leeuw R.: Folliculogenesis in hypophysectomised rats after treatment with recombinant human follicle-stimulating hormone. *Biol Reprod.*, 51:72-81, 1994.
17. Uilenbroek J.T., Kramer P., Karels B., de Jong F.H.: Significance of oestradiol for follicular development in hypogonadotropic immature rats treated with FSH and hCG. *J. Reprod. Fertil.*, 110(2):231-236, 1997.
18. The European Recombinant Human LH Study Group (1988): Recombinant human luteinising hormone (LH) to support recombinant human follicle stimulating hormone (FSH)-induced follicular development in LH- and FSH-deficient anovulatory women: a dose-finding study. *J. Clin. Endocrinol. Metab.*, 83, 5, 1507-1514.
19. Imthurn B., Macas E., Roselli M., Keller P.J.: Nuclear maturity and oocyte morphology after stimulation with highly purified follicle stimulating hormone compound and human menopausal gonadotropin. *Hum. Reprod.*, 11 (11):2387-2391, 1996.
20. Mercan R., Mayer J.F., Walker D., Jones S., Oehninger S., Toner J.P., Muasher S.J.: Improved oocyte quality is obtained with follicle stimulating hormone alone than with follicle stimulating hormone/human menopausal gonadotropin combination. *Hum. Reprod.*, 12(9):1886-1889, 1997.
21. Tornell J., Bergh C., Selleskog U., Hillensjo D.: Effect of recombinant human gonadotropins on oocyte meiosis and steroidogenesis in isolated

pre-ovulatory rat follicles. *Hum Reprod.*, 10(6):1619-1622, 1995.

22. Gordon U.D., Gordon A.C., Bonnar J., Harrison R.F.: Effect of differing doses of LH on oocyte maturation and fertilisation. Abstracts of the 13th Annual Meeting of the ESHRE, *Hum Reprod.*, p. 53, 1997.
23. Westergaard L.G., Erb K., Laursen S., Rasmussen P.E., Rex S.: The effect of human menopausal gonadotropin and highly purified, urine-derived follicle stimulating hormone on the outcome of in vitro fertilisation in down-regulated normogonadotropic women. *Hum. Reprod.*, 11(6):1209-1213, 1996.
24. Soderstrom-Antilla V., Tuija F., Hovatta O.: A randomised comparative study of purified follicle stimulating hormone and human menopausal gonadotropin for ovarian hyperstimulation in an oocyte donation programme. *Hum. Reprod.*, 11:1864-1870, 1996.
25. Fleming R., Chung C.C., Yates R.W.S., Coutts J.R.T.: Purified urinary follicle stimulating hormone induces different hormone profiles compared with menotropins, dependent upon the route of administration and endogenous luteinising hormone activity. *Hum. Reprod.*, 11:1854-1858, 1996.
26. Fleming R., Lloyd F., Herbert M., Fenwick J., Griffiths T., Murdoch A.: Effects of profound suppression of LH during controlled ovarian stimulation on follicular activity, oocyte and embryo function in cycles stimulated with purified FSH. *Hum. Reprod.*, 13(9):1788-1792, 1998.
27. Daya S., Gunby J., Hughes E.G., Collins J.A., Sagle M.A.: Randomised control trial of follicle stimulating hormone versus human menopausal gonadotropin in in-vitro fertilisation. *Hum. Reprod.*, 10(6):1392-1396, 1995.
28. Loumaye E., Vankjrieken L., Depresster S., Psalti I., de Coorman S., Thomas K.: Hormonal changes induced by short-term administration of a gonadotropin-releasing hormone agonist during ovarian stimulation for in vitro fertilisation and the consequences for embryo development. *Fertil. Steril.*, 51(1):105-111, 1989.
29. Tanbo T., Hhaug E., Dale P.O., Abyholm T., Kjekshus E.: Stimulation with human menopausal gonadotropin versus follicle stimulating hormone after pituitary suppression in polycystic ovarian syndrome. *Fertil. Steril.*, 53 (5):798-803, 1990.
30. Duijkers I.J.M., Vemer M., Hollanders J.M.G., Willemsen W.M.P., Bastiaans L.A., Hamilton C.J.C.M., Thomas C.M.G., Borm G.F.: Different follicle stimulating hormone - luteinising hormone ratios for ovarian stimulation. *Hum. Reprod.*, 8(9):1387-1391, 1993.
31. Sills E.S., Schattman G.L., Veeck L.L., Liu H.C., Prasad M., Rosenwaks Z.: Characteristics of consecutive in vitro fertilisation cycles among patients treated with follicle stimulating hormone (FSH) and human menopausal

gonadotropin versus FSH alone. *Fertil. Steril.*, 69(5):831-835, 1998.
32. Weston A.M., Zelinski-Wooten M.B., Stouffer R.L., Wolf D.P.: Developmental potential of embryos produced by in vitro fertilisation from gonadotropin-releasing hormone antagonist treated macaques stimulated with recombinant human follicle stimulating hormone alone or in combination with luteinising hormone. *Hum. Reprod.*, 11(3):608-613, 1996.
33. Rekha P., Mowat L., Jamieson M.E., Yates R.W., Fleming R.: Effect of profound suppression of luteinising hormone during treatment with gonadotropin releasing hormone analogue and purified follicle stimulating hormone upon development of cryopreserved embryos. *Hum. Reprod.*, 13 (3):696-698, 1998.
34. Gordon U.D.: *Evaluation of the role of luteinising hormone in ovarian steroidogenesis and follicular maturation.* MD thesis. Trinity College Dublin.
35. Hull M.G.R., Corrigan E., Piazzi A., Loumaye E.: Recombinant human luteinising hormone: an effective new gonadotropin preparation. *Lancet*, 344(8918):334-335, 1994.
36. Kousta E., White D.M., Piazzi A., Loumaye E., Franks S.: Successful induction of ovulation and completed pregnancy using recombinant human luteinising hormone and follicle-stimulating hormone in a woman with Kallmann's Syndrome. *Hum. Reprod.*, 11(1):70-71, 1996.
37. Zelinski-Wooten M.B., Hess D.L., Wolf D.P., Stouffer R.L.: Steroid reduction during ovarian stimulation impairs oocyte fertilisation, but not folliculogenesis, in rhesus monkeys. *Fertil. Steril.*, 61:1147-1155, 1994.
38. Reshef E., Lei Z.M., Rau C.H.V., Chegnini N., Luborsky J.L.: The presence of gonadotropin receptors in non-pregnant uterus, human placenta, fetal membranes and decidua. *J. Clin. Endocrinol. Metab.*, 70:421-430, 1990.
39. Li T.C., Serle E., Warren M.A., Cooke I.D.: Is endometrial development in the peri-implantation period influenced by high concentrations of luteinising hormone in the follicular phase ? *Hum. Reprod.*, 8(7):1021-1024, 1993.